Meditation Made Easy

Meditation Made Easy

LORIN ROCHE, Ph.D.

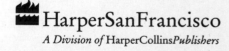

HarperSanFrancisco
A Division of HarperCollinsPublishers

Illustrations by Richard Kinsey

MEDITATION MADE EASY. Copyright © 1998 by Lorin Roche, Ph.D.
All rights reserved. Printed in the United States of America. No part of this book
may be used or reproduced in any manner whatsoever without written permission
except in the case of brief quotations embodied in critical articles and reviews.
For information address HarperCollins Publishers, Inc., 10 East 53rd Street,
New York, NY 10022.

HarperCollins Web Site: http://www.harpercollins.com

HarperCollins®, ▦ ®, and HarperSanFrancisco™ are trademarks of
HarperCollins Publishers Inc.

HarperCollins books may be purchased for educational, business, or sales
promotional use. For information please write: Special Markets Department,
HarperCollins Publishers, Inc., 10 East 53rd Street, New York, NY 10022.

FIRST EDITION

Design by Helene Wald Berinsky

Library of Congress Cataloging-in-Publication Data
Roche, Lorin
    Meditation made easy / Lorin Roche : illustrations by Richard Kinsey.
—1st ed.
        p.   cm.
    ISBN 0–06–251542–X (pbk.)
    1. Meditation.   I. Title
BL627.R613   1998   98-22600
158.1'2—dc21

    00 01 02 ❖/RRD(H) 10 9

To Those Who Make the Path by Walking It

To All Who Have Ever Walked Point

To the Search & Rescue Teams of All Time

CONTENTS

Meditation ◎◎◎ ◎◎◎ Made Easy

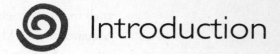 Introduction

Have You Ever . . .

- Drifted slowly awake and lain there in a delicious restfulness for a few moments before opening your eyes?

- Looked at the night sky and felt utter wonder at the vastness?

- Merged so deeply with the melody and rhythm of music you love that your sense of self disappeared in the ocean of sound?

- Felt electricity coursing through your body when you made love? At the moment of orgasm, been filled with brilliance or fireworks? Or in the afterglow, felt your body shimmering and pulsing with a vibrant peace?

- Inhaled a smell so delicious, perhaps your favorite dish when you were really hungry, that you almost swooned?

- Sat by a river, conscious of its steady flow, and entered into a sense of stillness?

- Been so in love that your heart seemed to turn to light?

. . . Then you have already experienced meditative awareness. These are all spontaneous experiences, typically lasting from a few seconds to a few minutes. Attention expands beyond its confines and touches something greater, something of the essence of life. Human beings have been experiencing these sorts of things since before there was the language to speak of them.

Meditative experience is no different from these naturally occurring moments. It is just intentional. What I am calling a "meditation technique" is paying attention to the rhythm of such an experience, tracking it through all its phases, and returning again and again to be educated by it. Most of what is meant by "practicing meditation" is just spending time being in the presence of such a quality of attention, then enjoying the effect on your daily life. Meditation is the practice of developing your capacity for rich experience.

Each of us is a yogi for half a second when we stop to smell the roses. It's all there in that moment of conscious, grateful breathing. When we cultivate our gratitude for breath, something good happens at a deep level. We make friends with life.

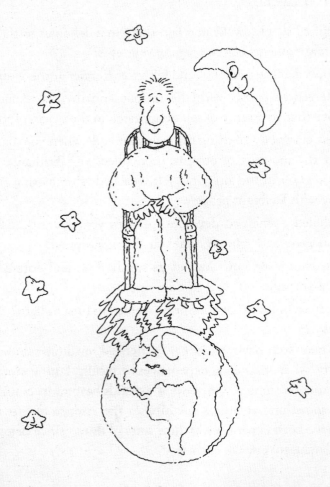

Welcome

Something has led you to be interested in meditation—your curiosity, your desire to explore, a longing for a little rest and relaxation, or the recommendation of a friend or doctor. Well, come on in.

Meditation is a great gift to give yourself. It is a way to experience a higher quality of life just by going inside yourself and touching your center for a moment. It is a brief retreat from the world that lets you reenter the world with a more vivid presence.

If you have never meditated before, this book will be your guide to some of the simplest and most widely practiced meditations in the Western world. They are all simple techniques you can do on your own; they involve things like paying attention to your breathing, listening to quiet sounds, and tracking the movement of your thoughts. You can start by doing the exercises for one or two minutes at a time, and as you grow more skillful you can meditate longer.

If you have meditated before, you probably started and stopped a number of times, looking for ways of practicing that suited your individual nature and lifestyle. You may have learned a technique from a friend, a teacher, or a class that did not suit you. Perhaps it was like a shoe that doesn't quite fit—okay to try on in the store but uncomfortable to walk in. My approach is about taking what usually seem like obstacles to meditation—your busy mind, your long days, your desires—and making them into your allies.

You will find the exercises in this book useful for getting started again and for learning how to customize your meditation to your needs. You also may find that the exercises help your meditation become easier, more restful, and more interesting.

This is come-as-you-are meditation. You do not have to be other than you are to begin. There are no impossible-to-do techniques, no uncomfortable postures, no onerous rules to follow.

If you invest the time in exploring how your individual nature interacts with these techniques, you will likely develop some powerful tools to enhance your life. The work for you is to engage your curiosity and sense of adventure. The rewards are a greater ability to pay attention to life and to love.

Almost everything we think of as meditation is flavored slightly with the view from behind the monastery walls. The ideas that in meditation you are supposed to *sit still and make your mind empty, aspire to high spiritual ideals, override or kill the ego,* and *cultivate detachment* from things—all these come from the spiritual tradition for recluses. They may be wisdom if you are a monastic, but they are poison if you live in the world. These are not general truths any more than the rules for Ping-Pong are universal, applying to tennis, golf, volleyball, baseball, and every other sport.

Meditation is about being intimate with your deepest self. Any sense of formality, any sense that you are doing a technique that comes from outside yourself interferes with this necessary closeness.

Meditation can and should be something that you reach for as informally as you reach for a cup of tea, or an apple, or the phone to talk to a friend—in other words, as a direct response to sensing some need in your body or heart. Meditation can be something you look forward to after you roll out of bed in the morning, to help you wake up and get ready for the day. It is something you may find yourself wanting to do when you walk in the door after work, to unwind and revitalize yourself. It is not really that meditation is "better" than sitting on the sofa and having a glass of wine while listening to music on the stereo. Meditation is just as much fun, but it provides more relief, works better, and is cheaper. Taking this informal approach to being with yourself will help you keep meditation simple, a simple pleasure and a relief.

Approaching meditation as a pleasurable indulgence will help you develop good instincts for your path, because instinctive guidance comes from the same place as your cravings and desires. You will need to be in touch with your instincts because you are your own guide in meditation, with your own daily life as your feedback mechanism.

Your instincts do not necessarily feel "spiritual." Far from it—they feel down-home, selfish, and spontaneous. The instincts are seat-of-the-pants and gut feelings. And they are often the first thing that gets thrown overboard when people try to be spiritual. But they are the essence of spirituality. They represent deep wisdom. The instincts move us to explore the world, survive, thrive, communicate, bond, reproduce, and rejoice. The urge to explore meditation is just as instinctive as the urges to talk to other people, work to assure your survival, explore your sexuality, and party. Spirituality is a spontaneous alchemy that occurs when all the instincts are working together. This happens only when all of human nature is embraced.

Meditation is not one monotone mood of reverence, nor is it only irreverence. It is a wide-open embrace of every possible mood, emotion, and current of your being: that is its simplicity and its challenge. Therefore I advocate a radical informality with the self as the essence of the approach to meditation. In an informal approach, the rebel in you is just as important as the sincere seeker. The impulse that says *Uh, I don't want to meditate today* is just as useful and informative as the impulse that says *I really want and need to meditate. I have an important day.*

For those of us who work hard and barely have enough real time for ourselves and our families, meditation can be incredibly useful: creating stronger, more resilient health and more consistent energy; helping us to be more at ease and perceptive in our relationships; and opening entire new worlds of gratitude, wonder, and well-being. Meditation should fit into our lifestyle naturally. In this book you will learn how to adapt your practice to the changing conditions of your life.

If you live in the world and work long days, you already crave stillness and rest; this is not something that has to be imposed from On High. This craving is called "wanting a vacation"—and you achieve it by giving in to the craving. Meditation is the practice of giving in to such cravings and letting them carry us into our interior worlds. This feels like an indulgence; indeed, the sense of luxury is one of the ways of knowing you are doing it right. Meditation is powered by our deepest cravings, not by discipline.

No one with a busy life can or should try to empty the mind, whatever that means. It is not that in meditation you won't find yourself sitting very still and going to a place beyond ordinary thought; it's just that any attempt to impose this on yourself will backfire. Imposition just makes a person more restless. Meditation for people who live in the world should strengthen the ego and enliven the connection to

Make Meditation a Mini-Vacation

the fires of passion. The more you embrace your passion, the more readily you will go beyond it to places of total repose inside yourself.

Meditation is quietly sexy, in the way that getting a massage or listening to great music is. The subtle currents of electricity that flow sweetly through the body, touching you everywhere, are to be cherished. Meditation allows the body to tune itself up to be ready for work, play, sleep, and all the exquisite pleasures of life. Let's say you walk in the door from work and you have half an hour to prepare yourself to be intimate with the one you love. What do you do? If you know how to meditate you would certainly spend some time that way, for one of the greatest gifts of meditation is that of enabling you to be completely present with sensuous experience, open to life with your senses shimmering, with a quality of surprise and novelty.

Food is best appreciated by those who have had an active day and built up a good appetite. Water is loved the most by people who have been out in the sun working up a sweat and come in to drink a refreshing glass. Meditation is best known by the people who need it most, who are out there in life putting their plans, desires, and ambitions into action. It should have a sense of luxury and deliciousness. It should be a place for you to entertain all your desires and longings and prepare to fulfill them as much as is possible and ethical in your life. If you lose track of your deepest desires and longings, then what will be your anchor? The idea that you should give up or distance yourself from your desires and your ego in meditation is nonsense. When people succeed in relinquishing desire, they tend to lose vitality.

You want meditation to be in the service of a better relationship with yourself and the world. This means having a more lively channel between your inner resources of love, passion, generosity, and curiosity and your outer life and relationships, where all those qualities are needed. The meditations presented in this book are all simple sensory-alertness exercises that will help you to have a more appreciative grasp of your everyday life.

Longing is your best clue to what is good for you. You will have to work at investigating your longings. Go into them deeply and find out what you really want most passionately. Engaging with your hankerings, lusts, desires, and longings will take you straight into your heart, not hell. If you love music of any kind, you already know much about your longings—just notice what is awakened in your body when you listen to what you love with complete abandon. Notice what kinds of music you crave and when. The same instinct you use to choose what music to play will guide you in selecting what meditations to do.

Be safe on your journey. Safety comes from being alert and relaxed as you move through your life. Let your best instincts guide you. Be awake to beauty. Be merciful to yourself and others. Cultivate your desires and enthusiasm for life. Meditation is enthusiasm for the simple: the simplicity of breath flowing in and out of us, day and night, for as long as we live.

My Story

I was five years old the first time I saw someone meditate. One morning I went into the living room to watch cartoons on television. As I entered the room, there in one of the big comfortable chairs was my uncle Bud, absorbed in reading a book.

After the cartoons were over, I turned off the television and saw Bud sitting there with his eyes closed, glowing with peacefulness. I had never seen an adult sit so still and be so at home in himself. He was as comfortable as a baby sleeping, and as powerful as a father. In my young life, I had never encountered those two things occurring in the same body.

I immediately went over to him and asked, "What are you doing?"

"Well, I *was* meditating," Bud said, opening his eyes.

"What's that?" I asked.

To his eternal credit, Bud did not look at me with irritation. He had a twinkle in his eyes as he said, "I am reading this book here." He pointed to a thick blue book on the table next to him. "And one of the things it says to do is to meditate." My mind went silent at that moment. I looked at him, then ran off to play with my favorite toy truck.

That is all I ever heard about meditation until thirteen years later.

It was 1968 and I was a freshman at the University of California's new campus at Irvine. Because it was a new campus, the researchers were desperate for human subjects. They made it a rule that all social science majors had to participate in many hours of experiments as part of our course requirements. I signed up for three weeks of afternoons in a lab that was doing research on brain waves.

When I showed up, I learned that my role in the research was to sit in an overstuffed chair in a soundproof room in total darkness, doing nothing for two and a half hours. By the flip of a coin, I had been selected as a "control" subject, which meant that I received no instructions on what to do in there.

At first I was disappointed, because the other subjects were getting brain-wave biofeedback, and that sounded interesting. I knew absolutely nothing about meditation or any other mental technique, so I just sat in the dark. To my great surprise, I found myself becoming extremely relaxed. All my senses opened up wide to the darkness and silence. It was incredibly luxurious.

When I came out of the lab, colors were very bright and everything seemed vivid and beautiful. I found I could do my calculus homework in less time than usual, and writing essays for literature class was much easier. My mind worked like a finely tuned machine and my body felt fantastic from the intense relaxation. Whatever I wanted to pay attention to, my mind would stay in tremendous alertness. Rather than taking hours out of my day, the afternoons in the lab seemed to give me extra time for life.

After the experiment ended, I missed having the quiet time. So I started sitting in a darkened room with my eyes closed and my ears plugged. One day a few weeks later a woman on the research team showed me a little paperback book she was reading. It was *Zen Flesh, Zen Bones*, by Paul Reps (it is still in print and currently published by Shambhala). I opened it to the back, to a chapter named "Centering," and saw a list of a hundred or so classical meditation techniques. This chapter was a translation of a four-thousand-year-old Sanskrit text called the Bhairava Tantra. Reading through the list of techniques, I felt my whole body tingle because I had experienced many of them spontaneously sitting in the lab. The Bhairava Tantra became my guide and I kept the book with me for years. Somehow I still have that original copy, although its pages have come loose. It is my Velveteen Rabbit. It is worn out from being loved.

Because I needed a job, I wound up working in that lab as a research assistant. Part of my job was to train people in basic meditation techniques and then measure the effect on their brain waves. This led to my becoming a full-fledged meditation teacher. Over the last thirty years I have worked with thousands of people in many settings—in homes, businesses, hospitals, homeless shelters, mountain retreats, and island resorts. I have found that meditation can be joyful and spontaneous for most people. It is this experience I share with you in this little book. You will have your own way of learning that is different from anyone else's. Have fun with meditation. Let it be a useful and beneficial experience. Go ahead, explore.

How to Use This Book

HOW TO READ THIS BOOK

You could read a thousand books on meditation and if you didn't experiment, didn't jump in and get your feet wet, you would never know how to do it. The way to learn a skill so it becomes part of your muscle memory is to learn one bit of information, then practice it right away. So I recommend that as you read this book, you pause every once in a while just to let the information sink in.

This book is designed to be read a few pages a day, just before and after you meditate. Of course, you can explore it any way that suits you. Feel free to dive in and read it from cover to cover. Or flip through and let whatever catches your eye define your reading for the day.

No matter what your style is, make sure you are comfortable and not reading with a furrowed brow. Also see that the space around you feels good. It's okay to read in bed, in a messy office, on an airplane . . . but if you can, take charge and arrange your environment to be as beautiful (whatever that means to you) as possible. It's best to read where you plan to meditate. It will become an easy ritual for getting into your meditation each day.

DEVELOPING YOUR OWN STYLE OF READING

Here are a few more suggestions to help you get started.

Read in your usual style, at your usual speed. Whether that means moving from the beginning of the book to the end fairly quickly or proceeding slowly and carefully, go right ahead. Maybe you'll read a little, then stop to do a meditation exercise here and there. Or perhaps you like to read some text, underline things, and jot down notes in a journal; that's fine, too. You've read a lot of books in your life. You know how.

OR

You could change your reading style radically, just for the fun of it. For example, you could slow down your reading speed, reflecting on one page at a time and really savoring it. You could develop a "meditative style" of reading. If you are feeling intuitive today, you might know exactly what page you want to turn to and how you want to shape your time.

Remember, every day your style can and will change, and that is fine.

MEDITATIVE READING

What's a meditative style of reading? It's really simple—just pause at the end of each paragraph or each page and take a couple of conscious breaths. (This pause is actually a mini-meditation, and all you have to do is breathe.) If you want to, shift your gaze from the book right out the window and rest it on a cloud or a colored rooftop; or close your eyes gently and breathe. Enjoy the experience of air flowing in and out as you process the information you've just covered. This will help you translate the information in the book into an internal ability.

Although meditative reading requires only a few seconds, it will probably take some getting used to. Its benefit is that it gives your body a chance to inwardly practice meditative awareness.

How to Combine Meditating and Reading

- Read and then meditate. That is, leisurely read two or three pages of this book in a sitting, then practice a few minutes of meditation, then call it a day. You might do that for the first month.

- Head right to the section called "Getting In" or to the "Getting into Breath" section. Select one of the meditations and do it for five minutes.

- Read and do mini-breathing meditations: do a five-second meditation at the end of each paragraph. Pause and take a conscious breath. Then move on. As you get used to the idea of this, you may sometimes slip into a pleasurable breath meditation and decide to stop reading for a while.

You can experiment with this right now. Right now as you are reading these words, breathe in just a tiny bit more deeply than usual. Notice the sound you make. Somewhere in the air's journey through the nose, sliding softly down the throat, gently filling the lungs, your body expands subtly to accept the air. Notice the little pause at the end of the inhalation as the breath turns to flow out. Somewhere in there you will discover a place of pleasure and restfulness. Notice what it's like. Remember this feeling and revisit it when you do your mini-breathing meditations.

If you feel comfortable with one breath, add a few more. Keep going until you spend one full minute with your breathing. It may feel like loafing, and that's good. Try it; see if you like it. Doing this may change your whole experience of reading the book—it may make it seem as if you are learning from your breath more than you are learning from the words on the page. That's good, too.

If this were a cookbook, you could read it in the kitchen, perhaps with it open on the counter, as you experimented with proportions and spices. If it were a book on tennis, you could look at illustrations of how to grasp the racket, and then you could grab your racket and put your hands around it. These would be ways of practicing what you had just read.

> **Tip:** One breath is the basic unit of learning in meditation. Three breaths is the beginning of a cycle of going into meditation. Most of what you learn about meditation will happen because you stay with an experience for fifteen seconds or longer, instead of five. When you take a few conscious breaths after reading something, you shift your sensory focus from words to feeling your body. When you do this, your body gets to assimilate the learning.

Since this is a meditation book, one way to practice what you read is to do a short meditation, anywhere from five seconds to a minute, anytime you find something that you want to make part of your instinctive learning.

HOW MUCH SHOULD I READ?

To begin, read and meditate less than you want. The most important thing is that you do not feel that there's a struggle to be undergone or a chore to be done. The best feeling is one of not really doing anything. That's what "effortless" is.

I suggest you spend, at most, thirty minutes a day with the book. Consider spending about ten minutes actually reading—anywhere from two to ten pages a day. Then do one of the meditations for maybe five or ten minutes. Spend the rest of the time resting. That's it.

Sensuous Reading

You may create a more luxurious way of reading if you wish. Choose a special time to do your reading and meditating. Sit down with this book right when you are on the edge of meditating, when you are just about to go in or come out. Make sure that it's a time when you really want to relax and soak into the essence of yourself. Think of it as a time to indulge, not study. This attitude will create a very sensual, smooth way of learning. Enjoy.

To enhance your mood, take a bath right before you begin, light a candle or incense, make a fire, or do whatever you need to do to make your environment especially inviting.

Other Ways of Focusing

As you read, you can place your attention on any number of things to help you feel more grounded, more secure, more focused.

- Feel the ground beneath you. Settle into gravity as it attracts you to the Earth's center. Give thanks to gravity for keeping you on the ground. Take delight in the simple relief of closing the eyes for a moment. Notice what it feels like to blink, and let the eyelids stay closed for a second or two longer. . . . Ahhh.

- Stretch often while reading, and notice how good it feels. Welcome your impulse to move. There's no need to get into a struggle with movement.

- When thoughts come, or melodies go through your head, be glad for them. Your attention will come back to the book automatically. Don't worry.

- Pause and savor the insights, ideas, pictures, or sensations you have while reading. Think of them as gifts, not distractions.

Developing a Healthy Attitude Toward Meditation

I want you to develop a relationship with meditation that is healthy—as healthy as the best stuff you've got going in your life. You know what those things are. Everyone has a healthy relationship with something: music, dance, novels, theater, dogs, horses, poetry, food, sports, driving, starting businesses, friends. Healthy relationships evolve gradually. They grow and blossom over time. Your appreciation and understanding of meditation mirror that path. Your purpose the first few weeks is simply to get comfortable with meditation and have a good time. Meditate less than you want to, and look forward to the next time you get to sit down (or stand or lie down) and practice. Looking forward to meditating is an important part of learning. It's like a date. It can be wonderful, fun, relaxing, comfortable, something you want to do if it's right.

Maybe your best way of developing your relationship with meditation and with yourself is to have a date with yourself each evening—an appointment to meditate. Just show up and be with yourself, and get used to having a special quiet time.

Try not to be competitive with yourself. There is no need to impose meditating past the point of comfort. One-minute meditations are the stuff

> **Tip:** Meditation is an unusual skill in that you learn it by resting. That is the practice: resting in yourself with attention. You learn meditation by doing exactly the kind of things that got you in trouble at school: looking out the window and daydreaming, or closing your eyes and drifting off. As you read this book, the more you drift off and make your own associations, the better.

longer meditations are made of. The advantage of meditating for one or two minutes is that you won't have a chance to develop the attitude of trying or making an inappropriate effort. Meditation should never require any more effort than reading your favorite book or listening to your favorite music.

Making an effort is the only thing you have to be concerned about avoiding. A healthy attitude toward meditation is nonrepressive, non-controlling, nonaggressive. It is restful, easy, and free. It is much more important to develop this type of approach than to spend a certain number of minutes meditating.

How to Select Which Meditation to Do

- Simply explore whatever meditations appeal to you and give you pleasure. In the first few weeks you might want to read "Questions and Answers," then select one of the techniques in "Getting into Breath" or "Getting into Sound" and make friends with it.

- Use the same sensibility for choosing a meditation that you use for shopping or for selecting music to listen to, clothes to wear, and books to read. This is your hunting-and-gathering instinct. You need only find one or two meditation techniques to keep you going for several months or even years!

- Jump right into the "Obstacles" section. That's a good way to understand some of the things that might get in the way of your meditating and to find out how to deal with them. If you are a worrier, that section is a good place to hang out.

- Read the "Getting In" section several times, and then do the Do Nothing technique.

- If you are feeling "sensual," do the Salute the Senses technique or the Feeling at Home exercise. Then start to explore the Mini-Meditations.

- Trust yourself. You'll know what you need to do. Really.

- Keep yourself interested. Don't let yourself be bored. Move on if you want more. Stay with any meditation you love until you're satisfied. Think of it as food for your soul, and eat when you are hungry.

When in Doubt

If you are meditating and an experience comes up that you do not know how to handle, stop meditating and turn to the "Obstacles" section. It's your first-aid kit. Don't worry; anything and everything you might wonder about is covered in the Obstacles section—from thinking you have too many thoughts to trouble with noise, from emotions that are coming up to weird body sensations.

Tip: *Whenever you come across something you want to know, reread it a few times. It takes a while to sink in. After reading it, close your eyes and pay attention to your breathing for a minute. That will let the learning settle into your nerves and reflexes. Meditation is more like a sport than a mental skill.*

The time you give to meditation, it will give back to you. I have consistently found that meditation gives me back more time than I give it. You'll know you have been meditating because you are more relaxed as you go through your day and night.

Always keep in mind that meditation is very simple. All you have to do is breathe. Your body will go into and out of meditation spontaneously. It can feel like a conscious nap. Read at your own pace and explore meditation at your own pace. We are all different in our learning styles and speed. Honor your own individualistic way of learning as you explore the exercises in this book.

Introducing a little meditation in your life can be as simple as taking time to watch the sunrise—not just for a two-second glance but for minutes. It can be as simple as taking a full minute of breathing in the delicious smell of your food before you begin eating.

☺ Questions and Answers

What Is Meditation?

Meditation is a naturally occurring rest state; it is resting in yourself while remaining awake and alert. Meditation is innate, and your body already knows how to do it. The human body has an instinctive ability to shift into profound rest states in order to heal, energize, integrate, tune itself up, and assimilate learning. It is almost a sure bet that you have already experienced this many times in your life.

Meditation is paradoxical in that you are resting more deeply than you do in sleep, yet you are wide awake inside. It is very similar to taking a nap, but you don't fall asleep—you fall awake. You can induce this state by attentively doing anything simple and repetitive. We breathe all the time, and breathing is rhythmic, so you could pay attention to your breathing. There are so many ways in.

Meditation promotes a heightened awareness of the details of everyday life. Even a few minutes of meditation will help you move through the world with more relaxation and alertness.

Meditation is giving attention a chance to explore its full range, both inward and outward. It is a conversation between your inner and your outer life. This sounds simple, and it is. But there is no end to the delights of attention; there is always more to learn, more to explore, more to awaken to.

Where Did Meditation Come From?

Meditation was probably discovered independently by hunters, singers, dancers, drummers, lovers, and hermits, each in their own way. People tend to encounter meditative states whenever they throw themselves with total intensity into life's callings. The knowledge of how to intentionally cultivate meditative states is a kind of craft knowledge—those handy tips people pass on to each other. Meditation does not come from India or Tibet—those are just places where the knowledge rested for a while, and the hermits in those places wrote it all down. Bless them.

Human beings have been using tools for hundreds of thousands of years, according to the archaeologists. I consider it very likely that they have been using sophisticated mental tools for tens of thousands of years.

Hunters, for example, sometimes have to make themselves still for hours. They have to merge with the forest and not even think, lest they scare the prey away. Then they leap into action with total precision at a moment's notice—that's Zen in a nutshell. Hunters teach each other these skills, through verbal instruction and example.

Singers and dancers often enter meditative states through their passionate expression. Singers work with breath awareness in ways far more sophisticated than yoga. Lovers are often in a state of heightened appreciation that borders on meditation. Hermits are the ones we have heard the most from, because they kept the best notes. That is why we always think of yogis and bearded guys in the Himalayas when we think of meditation. But their way is only one small subset of the many different gateways into meditation.

Meditation comes from the human heart and is a way of warming your hands and your life at the fire always pulsing there in your core. It comes from the depths of your instinctive wisdom. Human beings are always wondering and inquiring, and meditation is a natural emergence of that adventure.

On the other hand, cats obviously meditate. That's what it looks like to me, anyway. So it may be a genetically encoded, instinctive talent in mammals. Cats don't need to be taught to meditate, but human beings need a little coaching.

Why Do People Meditate?

People meditate for innumerable reasons, and all of them are valid. Here are a few:

- People meditate out of curiosity, wonder, and a desire to explore.
- People meditate because they are worried, tired, bored, lonely, horny, or tense.
- People meditate because they are happy, grateful, in love, streaming with delight, and glad to be alive.
- People meditate because they are grieving, sad, despairing, resigned, frustrated.
- People meditate because they have lost someone or some part of themselves or lost the joy of life.
- People meditate because they feel out of place in the world created by human beings and prefer to live in the world of Nature.
- People meditate as an attempt to escape from life and from Nature.
- People meditate because they are sick in body or soul and need healing.

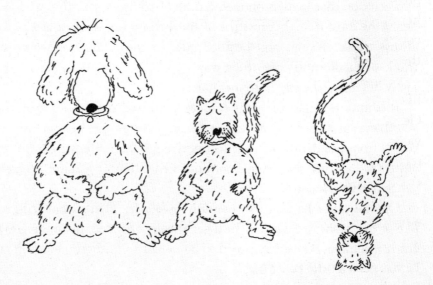

- People meditate because they feel perfectly at home and want to savor the feeling.

- People meditate to touch the essence of life and bring its magic into everyday living.

- People meditate because they have not touched the essence of life but suspect that it is there for the touching.

- People meditate because it is an urge in them that they have long felt, and it gradually condensed into a movement they realize is meditation.

- People meditate as a response to the calling of their own souls.

- People meditate because they are so excited by life they figure they could use a little calmness.

- People meditate to keep their intuition and senses sharp.

Each of these impulses has generated a variety of techniques and traditions. Honor them in yourself, as they come and go. And whenever you read or hear something about meditation, you can wonder, which emotion does this emerge from?

It is always good to take a moment and feel what it is you want out of meditation, what impulses are moving you. That is part of the preparation for meditation. The list above is by no means comprehensive—make your own list. Your list can be a description of how you want to feel, or the practical outcome you want, or a mingling of the two.

Meditation is there to help you fulfill your everyday needs. Things like getting a little rest and relaxation. Clearing your mind of clutter. Getting some perspective on your life, as you would if you were on vacation. Having more energy. Being able to go into action with relaxation, even if you're facing a test, an interview, or some other crucial action.

The key is to know what you want, or at least be open to what you want out of meditation. That is the passion that will lead you to invest time in meditation. Then, the moment you enter meditation, let go completely of your expectations.

Why Should I Meditate?

During meditation we can rest more deeply than in sleep, yet the mind is free to think deeply about what is going on in our lives and to come up with a new perspective. Often what we have perceived as a threat is downgraded to just a challenge or "something interesting on the horizon." The nerves can stop their emergency functioning. Or it could be the opposite: we might have been missing the real urgency of a situation because we were flooded with distracting details. In either case, meditation promotes the ability to be relaxed and focused while engaged in action, and to get tense only when it is absolutely necessary.

Even a few minutes of meditation can help you shift gears at the end of the day, from work mode to being-with-the-family mode or play mode. In the morning, a few minutes of meditation can help you feel more alert and relaxed all day.

Because most human illnesses are caused by or worsened by stress, meditation is good for your health. A lot of problems in relationships are caused by one or both partners being under stress. Meditation helps relationships by giving you a way to release stress without dumping on your partner. Also, because in meditation you give yourself a lot of attention, you'll find you have more attention to give to other people. If you aren't as needy, and you can give as well as receive, all your relationships go a bit easier. Meditation is a kind of social lubricant.

The meditations in this book encourage greater adaptability, resilience, realistic appraisal of stress, emotional expressiveness, and appreciation of life's simple pleasures. What the path of meditation asks of you is steady inquiry into your own nature, which is something you are doing anyway—it's called having desires.

I Don't Have Time for This, What Do I Do?

You can meditate for one minute here, three minutes there. Properly done, meditation always gives you more time than it takes.

As you learn to love meditation, you will create more time for it.

The busier your life is, the more you crave a vacation. That wanting-a-vacation feeling is one of the main reasons people meditate, and it is a gateway right on in. People who work hard want rest and renewal, and that is mainly what meditation is. Just don't make a big deal out of it, an impossible-to-achieve ideal.

Meditation can create the same feeling of relaxation and ease as going to a bar after work. The relaxation of meditation is what you would seek in a bar if you drink, in getting a massage if you could afford one each day, in going to Hawaii if you could somehow be transported there instantly after work. The most important thing is to approach meditation in the same natural way you would have a glass of wine, take a nap, listen to music, or go for a walk. Be completely unpretentious with yourself.

Can I Meditate Just Out of Curiosity?

Meditation is not just one sappy mood of reverence or quiet. It is a platform from which to witness all your moods. You can come as you are and meditate for any reason under the sun. You can meditate just to check it out; you can meditate in order to have better sex, or because you are stressed out, or because you want some enlightenment. You do not have to be "sincere" or "serious" to meditate. You could be making fun of the whole thing and still get a lot out of it.

Will I Need to Make Lifestyle Changes?

The meditation exercises in this book will probably not work well if you are using illegal drugs. Marijuana and psychedelics leave a kind of fog in the neurons that makes meditation seem boring, and these effects last for weeks.

Other than that, don't change anything unless you want to. Your lifestyle got you this far, so why change it now? You can smoke cigarettes, eat meat, drink coffee, have wine with dinner.

With regard to food, eat with gusto whatever makes you feel strong and energetic. In the long run, this will probably keep you healthier than following any particular set of rules.

If you are meditating as part of a health regimen or a "healthy heart" program, of course follow whatever suggestions the doctors have made. And if you are taking prescription medications, then keep taking them. Some people can reduce their blood pressure medication, for example, if they meditate consistently, but that is between them and their doctors.

Cherish your "vices," whatever they are; meditation will work its magic on your relationship with them. A lot of what are called vices are ways of letting off steam, releasing tension. When you are less tense, then you may find you don't need to do unhealthy things to unwind.

Do I Have to Sit Cross-Legged?

Sitting cross-legged works well for some people and it looks really cool. But this pose does nothing for meditation that can't be done in other ways. The main virtue of the cross-legged posture is that it's handy if you have no furniture, are homeless, or are outdoors.

Recently two yoga teachers came to me for meditation sessions in the same week. They were both lean young women, and they sat cross-legged on the floor during the session. They shifted around and had to

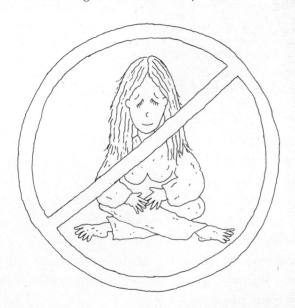

adjust their feet every few minutes. I didn't say anything at the time, because I just wanted to observe. But later I asked each of them and they admitted that they always sit in the cross-legged pose and their legs always hurt after a while when they do so.

On the other hand, or foot, I enjoy the cross-legged pose. It just feels nifty sometimes. I've used it about half the time in my thirty years of meditation.

If you can sit cross-legged with total comfort for half an hour without your feet going to sleep or getting uncomfortable—even a little— then go ahead. Remember, though, hurting your knees has nothing to do with getting enlightened.

Most of the meditations in this book are to be done sitting on a chair or sofa in your favorite place, or standing, walking, or lying down.

Don't I Have to Have a Guru?

No.

Do I Have to Sit Still?

What's stillness got to do with it? Move all you want in meditation. You only sit still in meditation to better follow the movement of life. It is a natural repose, not something forced.

When you are deeply absorbed in something—conversing, reading a book, listening to a piece of music—you will sometimes be very still. You become poised in order to better follow the flow of the conversation, the arc of the plot in the story, or the movement of the music. That is the way to be in meditation as well. So stillness of posture happens spontaneously; it is not something you focus on or make a rule out of.

Life is movement, an infinite dance on every level—atoms move and vibrate, cells undulate, blood pulses, breath flows, electrochemical impulses charge through your nerve pathways. If you are sitting while reading this book, your postural muscles are making lots of tiny little corrections to keep you upright, and the muscles in the diaphragm and ribs are moving with the gentle rhythm of respiration. Each of these little movements is part of the meditation experience.

The dance of life changes its pace according to whether we are walking, sitting very still, or lying down, but there is always a dance, always the hum and undulation of life.

When Should I Meditate?

You can meditate when you want to, or when you decide you should, or whenever you can sneak it in. It is up to you. The basic principle is to meditate before periods of activity, so that your ability to work and play and socialize can be enhanced by the relaxed alertness in which you are learning to function. The standard approach is to meditate soon after arising in the morning and then again before the evening meal. This works well for a lot of people, and it creates a beautiful feeling of rhythm to a day.

Other options are to meditate once a day in the afternoon or to have several mini-meditations throughout the day. If you meditate before sleep, keep it short and select meditations that are soothing.

How Long Should My Meditation Sessions Last?

Start with five minutes in the morning or in the evening. If that does not seem like enough time, then meditate for five minutes in the morning and again for five minutes in the evening. Later, when that does not seem like enough, increase your time little by little.

For the first month, the most important thing is to develop a sense of being at ease with yourself and having a good time. You could read this book for ten minutes or so, meditate for five minutes, and call it a day. Then come back tomorrow and continue. In the beginning, meditate less than you want to, so that you are always looking forward to the next session.

After a month, if ten minutes seems too short, then you can let yourself go a little longer. But do not meditate more than twenty minutes in the morning and in the evening until you have been at it for several years. It takes a long time to get used to being relaxed while in action, which is one of the main effects of meditation. There is a lot to learn about handling relaxation.

If you are really busy, even a few minutes of meditation is beneficial. There are lots of meditations in this book that require less than a minute, and they can be adjusted to last for anywhere from a few seconds to five minutes.

Where Should I Meditate?

Meditate wherever you are when you have the time. Some people meditate at their desks before leaving for lunch or at the end of the workday. If your schedule permits, pick a favorite spot in your house or garden or in nature to use for meditation. When I began meditating, I was a freshman in college with an intense study schedule and a job that took fifteen hours a week. I left the house early and came home late, so I used my car as a meditation spot in the late afternoons. There were lots of places to park that were under trees, in empty lots bordering on fields. I also meditated in churches and libraries. If you can arrange to have your own private spot, so much the better.

Pause Now and Take a Deep Breath

Pick spots that match your mood. Approach meditation as you would listening to music, if you love music. Be that informal and easy with yourself.

What Can I Do Wrong?

Working at it, trying, or forcing—that's almost the only thing you can do wrong in any meditation. If you are too carefree, it's easy to move in the direction of alertness when you want to. But if you are rushed or tense in your approach, you may build habits that prevent you from resting in meditation, and then you won't want to do it. Take a modified *hands-off* attitude toward your mind.

The Only Real Mistakes

- *Being unnatural with yourself in any way; leaving out or editing parts of yourself to fit into what you think "meditation" is. This includes trying to be spiritual. When you try to be spiritual, you edit out the parts that seem "unspiritual," such as sexuality, anger, jealousy, ambition, grief.*

- *Trying to control your experience.*

- *Trying to slow down.*

- *Not giving painful sensations a chance to resolve into relief.*

- *Depriving yourself of sleep.*

- *Being the Thought Police.*

These reminders are to help you educate your reflexes so that you cooperate with the process of meditation. They may seem obvious when you glance at them, but they are not obvious to meditators when they are learning. When you close your eyes, your experience is so immediate that you will respond more from reflex than from intuition.

Tip: Don't limit your range. Give yourself—your body—full permission to nod off or fall completely asleep, go silent, be very busy, have rapid thoughts, or become completely excited. It is typical for a meditator to range over time between comalike sleep (usually for twenty to forty minutes) while working off the sleep debt and times of incredible inner wakefulness. The nervous system is exercising its full range of motion and balancing itself.

This process takes place only to the extent that you feel safe. Any fear in your body blocks the process. This in itself is safe and self-regulating, because it avoids any sense that "something is happening to me." The fear keeps you from settling down deeper into meditation. Going step-by-step gradually dissolves the fear.

Meditation is a natural response of the human body. As with all natural movements, trying ruins the process. Trying to go to sleep, even if you are tired, can make you miserable. Trying to be sexually turned on to someone because you feel obligated to is disgusting. Trying to exercise when you don't want to is boring. Any sense of obligation or stuffiness kills the joy of it. If you find yourself taking meditation too seriously, rent your favorite comedy video and watch it for five minutes before doing the meditation exercises in this book.

What Do I Need to Get Started?

All you need are a comfortable chair, a couple of minutes, and one or more functioning sensory pathways, such as hearing or sight or touch. You can come in with any attitude you have: skepticism, curiosity, or enjoyment. Be willing to be surprised and energized, and be willing to fall asleep because you are so relaxed.

You do not need to know much to get started. Just treat meditation as if you were doing something you enjoy, such as listening to music, napping, drinking, eating, or reading. Put meditation into that slot in your life, with things you do to unwind or quietly have a good time. If you take this approach, you will discover connections between meditation and joyous indulgences you already know, and meditation will quickly become a treasured part of your daily life.

How Can I Accessorize for Meditation?

Clothing. Just wear whatever you are wearing—you can be comfortable or uncomfortable. Some of the best meditations I have ever had were while wearing a suit and a tie. I loosened the tie a little. Other all-time great meditations were when I was (1) naked, (2) wearing my favorite silk robe, (3) sitting on a rock wearing swimming trunks, (4) in bed, wrapped in a blanket. It is good to have a blanket or jacket handy in case you get chilled.

Chair. My favorite chair for meditating is a square waiting-room chair, the kind you see in doctors' offices. It is made of wood and has cloth over padding, and some padding on the arms. These chairs are stable and neither too soft nor too firm. If you sit upright in them, they offer just the right amount of back support. The chair supports your back up to about the middle, leaving the upper torso and head free to move. But you can sit on a sofa or on any comfortable chair anywhere you like. The main thing is that your feet touch the floor. If you are short, cut an inch or whatever is needed off the legs of the chair.

What Will Happen When I Meditate?

The main thing you will experience is rhythm, the continuous ebb and flow of many intersecting rhythms, because that is what life is. Your body and mind are composed of complex symphonies of rhythms.

The sensuous texture of meditation is infinitely varied: there are all kinds of subtle sensations, internal imagery, and sound effects. Experience changes moment-to-moment and is always sort of a surprise, like a good movie. One moment you will be in the bliss of an inner vacation, then suddenly you will be thinking of your laundry list. You will never have exactly the same experience twice.

In general, your experience will probably move among the following:

- Relaxation and relief.
- Sorting through thoughts about your daily life.
- Reviewing the emotions you felt during the day and giving them a chance to resolve.
- Brief moments of deep quiet and inner peace.
- Near-sleep and dreamlike images.
- Healing: reexperiencing and then letting go of old hurts.
- Tuning up: your nervous system fine-tuning itself to the optimal level of alertness.

Every thirty seconds or so, you will probably find your body shifting from one to another of these moods or modes.

You may feel relaxed during all these phases, but the aim of meditation is not relaxation. Meditation is an evolutionary instinct that works to make you more alert and capable of adapting after meditation.

Do I Have to Make My Mind Blank?

No, nor do you have to "empty your mind." This is a myth. There are moments of inner quiet, but thinking is a major part of meditation. You ride thoughts like surfers ride waves. The more you accept all thoughts, the more inner repose you will get.

Because the brain does a lot of sorting and housecleaning during meditation, it is often tremendously busy. The more your mind wanders during meditation, the more able it is to pay attention after meditation, because it has done its tuning-up.

Also, since you are relaxed during meditation, you learn to stay relaxed while thinking of things in your life that used to make you

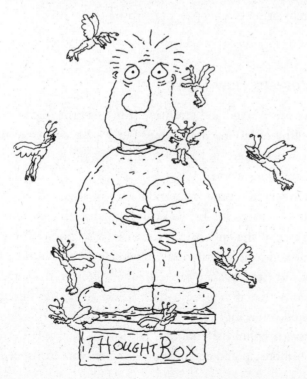

THOUGHTBOX

tense. You should expect your mind to be noisy part of the time in meditation. You won't care very much, though, because you will still be very relaxed. After meditation is when your mind will be quieter. And because your mind is quieter, those little thoughts you need to know can catch up with you. Your intuition, your gut feelings, your strategic overview, your hunches will emerge with greater clarity.

Do I Have to Concentrate?

People concentrate a great deal at work, so it would be redundant to concentrate during meditation. It would be a busman's holiday. In meditation you learn how to do the opposite of concentration; you learn to expand the scope of your attention. You learn a kind of attention that excludes nothing, and therefore the needy and unknown parts of yourself can come into range. This is what leads to integration of the personality and coordination of mind, heart, and body. Unlearning concentration is a big part of learning to meditate.

Do I Have to Slow Down?

When we are relaxed and attentive, time seems to open up, and there is the feeling of having more time. But we haven't slowed down—it's just that when there is less mental noise, we have a richer contact with the sensuous world.

Human reaction time is around a fifth of a second. If you see a herd of buffalo or cars racing by, you can recognize the situation and begin stepping out of the way in a fraction of a second. When someone is talking to you, you identify individual sounds in a hundredth of a second, because recognition time is much shorter than reaction time. That means that if you see a friend, you recognize her that quickly. Why would you want to slow down?

The truth behind the fantasy of slowing down is that meditation gives you more choice about your velocity: you can speed up or slow down as appropriate. Moreover, a synchronization of rhythms occurs during meditation that sometimes creates the feeling that there is more time in the day. Anyone can experience this—parents with their kids, athletes, drivers, musicians. When they are in their groove, they sometimes feel that there's a lot of time in a second. It comes about from heightened attentiveness.

So don't think you have to put on the brakes in order to meditate. Forget about controlling your speed during meditation. When a thought comes while you are meditating, you can identify what sort of thought it is earlier in the process of its development, because you are attentive. After meditation, there is typically a feeling of harmony, of moving through your day in sync with your inner rhythms. This creates the sense that there is more time in the day. You get to this experience by paying attention, not by trying to slow things down.

How Could Meditation Be "Easy"?

It is an illusion that there is some "oomph" that you need to apply to meditation, as if you have to push it or jump-start it. Meditation is not an old car with a dead battery. Meditation is recognizing and then giving in to your desire for rest, inner sanctuary, and relaxation. It's a relief to meditate once you know how. The fantasy of effort just gets in the way of meditation, in the same way that trying to go to sleep gets in the way of shifting from being awake to sleeping.

Most people wouldn't describe sitting on the sofa watching their favorite TV show as "hard." Then why would it be hard to close the eyes and watch the ongoing sitcom of your mind for half an hour? There might even be fewer commercials.

If you let meditation be a simple pleasure, it is easy to do. And if you meditate just for the joy of it, it will be good for you and self-reinforcing.

The amount of effort in meditation is about the same as that of listening to music you enjoy, especially if it's the kind you close your eyes to. Physiologically, meditation is a deeper rest than sleep, so it is by definition even easier than sleeping. The capacity to meditate is built in; you just need to trigger it, and this means allowing your body and mind to go into meditation.

Many things in life can be hard: finding someone to love is often hard; working out a relationship is hard; breaking up or staying together can be hard; jobs are hard. People dying is hard. You don't have to make meditation hard in order to create an aura of romance about it.

Is There Anything Difficult About Meditation?

Coming down off emergency functioning is hard. If you meditate after a stressful day during which you have been running on adrenaline, you'll feel pain for a while because your nerves are buzzing with stress. Sometimes meditation is that familiar pleasure-pain of resting when tired, and sometimes it is more pain than pleasure. Once I was meditating after a long, tiring day and was in the midst of feeling my nerves buzz with pain. I peeked at my watch to see what time it was, then went back to paying attention to the fatigue and pain. An hour later it seemed, I checked my watch again, and less than three minutes had gone by! Gradually, over minutes, as you pay attention, the sensation of tension turns into a pleasurable fatigue.

Meditation noticeably speeds up the process of shifting from emergency mode to pleasure mode, but you have to be willing to pay the price. The price is that you feel everything, every little buzz and ache in every nerve. The upside is that you feel a lot better after meditation. That's a huge upside, because it means you can walk into a room after a stressful day and walk out refreshed half an hour later. This has an immense impact on your life—you have your nerves back, you have your pleasure back, you have real energy instead of the false buzz of emergency. You won't need a glass of wine to relax, and when you eat dinner, you will actually taste your food instead of unconsciously gulping it. But this is the down-and-dirty, bottom-line nitty-gritty of meditation: are you willing to stay there and pay attention to your own healing?

Another thing that's hard is experiencing the deeper layers of your own healing. Anytime you are deeply relaxed and feeling safe, your brain will at some point bring up memories of past events when you felt unsafe and tense in order to erase the trauma and free the body of residual fear. To heal a painful memory, you have to relive it while in a safe and relaxed state. Often your brain will review a memory over and over until you can look at it and stay relaxed. This happens spontaneously during meditation, and it happens only to the extent that you can stay relaxed. This is a part of meditation that people have trouble with, because they don't understand it. On the other hand, pulling a thorn out of your foot hurts, but it's a lot easier than limping around, trying to avoid putting pressure on the part of your foot with the thorn in it.

Because you are relaxed in meditation, your residual tensions come to the surface to be reviewed, evaluated, and released. This same process goes on during sleep, but you are unconscious so you don't notice it. Meditation takes some of the load off sleep. If you have worked through the tensions of the day before going to bed, this tends to make sleep more restful and renewing.

What's a Meditation Technique?

The word *technique* comes to us from Latin and Greek words meaning "weave" and "texture." This is apt because in meditation you weave together all of who you are to pay attention to one thing.

There are two elements to any meditation technique: *how* you pay attention and *what* you pay attention to. The *how* is usually gentle, restful, steady attention, and the *what* is something simple yet sensuous and gorgeous—like breath. In meditation you rest attention in a sensory perception, take delight in it, then hang on for the ride.

Breath is an example of a sensual focus for meditation. Breath is infinitely interesting because it can be taken for granted, it can be frenzied, it can be passionate, it can be sweet, it can be energizing, and it can be soothing. Breath can wake you up and put you to sleep. Breath can be dignified and it can be wild. If you keep paying attention to breath, you will discover all these feelings in yourself. Breath is a love affair you are having with infinity, and the purpose of any meditation technique is to lead you into being a little bit more in love with life day by day.

There are thousands of meditation techniques, and all of them have been appropriate for someone, somewhere, at some time. The fact that the meditation traditions have preserved their records across thousands of years is one of the wonders of the world. Those records show that you can pay attention to almost anything as a meditation focus, if you really want to.

There are many subtle differences in the rules that each meditation tradition advocates, but these are just codifications of what worked in a given situation. They are not carved in stone. They are just rules, like the rules for rugby, soccer, football, tennis, and Ping-Pong. In all those games, there is a rectangular court and a ball. The rules are about what to do with that ball. You are allowed to hit the ball with your feet, head, hands, or a paddle. If meditation were a game, it would be to just let those thoughts sail on by, or over you, or under you. You win if you don't get caught up in trying to control them.

If you simply pay attention with a gentle, appreciative attitude and do not resist anything, you will tend to go into meditation right away. The body will just start to settle in. There is no need to control anything. Think of it as a conscious nap.

How Do I Know Which Technique to Do?

Use your shopping instinct—that's the modern-day equivalent of the hunting-gathering instinct. Follow your "hunches" and preferences as you do when you select music to listen to or television shows to watch. Use your natural curiosity and sense of exploration. It takes a little longer to find your own way in meditation, as opposed to having someone tell you what to do. But the exploring itself can be fun.

The purpose of any meditation technique is to lead you beyond the technique into a more immediate and vital contact with your everyday life. You will know, usually immediately, which techniques you like. They will be the ones that leave you feeling rested and more available for the joy of living.

Hey, you only need one or two meditation techniques to last you a year! But they have to be the right ones for you. Also, there is no One True Way to meditate. You can just do what works for you.

What's a Mantra and Do I Need One?

In Sanskrit, *mantra* literally means "a tool of thought." Sometimes, for some people, a mantra is a great tool to use in meditation.

Although there are many types of tools of thought—for example, visual images—in practice, the word *mantra* has come to mean thought as sound. Mantras are special sounds that are handy for use in meditation.

Shall I run that by you again?

Thoughts can come in any multimedia presentation—images, inner movies, abstract art, sounds, internal conversations, phrases, feelings, bodily sensations, even smells and tastes. When we are thinking, we think in combinations of all these. But because human language uses sound, and because people talk so much to one another, sound is a very useful meditation tool.

Right now, reading this book, you may be hearing the sounds of the words in a very abstract way inside yourself—not a clear enunciation.

You have already heard mantras many times in the euphonious sounds sung in church, temple, and chorale music. Alleluia. Hallelujah. Amen. Take one of those words and sing it right now, or chant it for a few minutes.

You have even made up mantras, or parts of them. Sounds such as "oh" and "ah" and "mmmmm," the kinds of sounds people naturally make when they are exclaiming, sighing, or expressing delight, are the components of mantras.

Some sounds generate a beautiful feeling that speaks to the body directly. You can listen to such sounds inwardly, without making any external sound, and the effect is like listening to internal music. It can be wonderfully restful. If you find a mantra you like and listen to it while meditating, it's as if the areas of the brain involved in speech are getting a massage.

Some people love to listen to mantras while meditating, and some people prefer things such as breath. As you explore the exercises, you can find out for yourself what your preferences are.

How Will I Know I'm Doing It Right?

If you are enjoying yourself, feel restful, and have a sense of ease, you are doing it right. In the long run, you know you are doing it right if you are more adaptable, resilient, and stable inside yourself and more perceptive and appreciative of life.

◉ Getting Started

Getting In

There are five stages of "getting in" to a meditation. While you are learning, linger in each stage for a while—a minute or two or more. Gradualness is everything in meditation. Once you get to know a meditation, you will glide from one stage to another spontaneously. Eventually, each stage can happen in seconds.

1. Set up the room.
2. Let background sensations come forward. Attend to inner needs.
3. Feel the call to meditate.
4. Match rhythms with yourself.
5. Include an opening ritual and statement of intention.

I. SET UP THE ROOM

First of all, check that the phone is off. If you live with people, tell them you are going to be meditating and not to come in, or put a note on the door. Don't tell them to be quiet, though. Noise is no problem. Check to make sure you have fresh air. If you will be meditating for more than five minutes, you might make sure there's a jacket, sweater, or blanket at hand in case you get cold. If you want to have a book of prayers, or a Bible, or poetry, put that by your spot.

Then look at the spot where you are going to sit and give yourself a chance to be attracted to it. I sometimes suggest to people that they stand near their spot until they really feel like sitting down. Don't make yourself sit.

2. LET BACKGROUND SENSATIONS COME FORWARD

The attitude of meditation is an open embrace of your entire being—who you are in your daily life and who you are in your inner self. It is because of this attitude that the outer and inner can meet, interact, and integrate.

You start by allowing background sensations, emotions, and thoughts to come to the surface and be tended to. The word *tender* is related to "attention" and that is what you do: you tender or pay attention to yourself. You begin this process before you close your eyes simply by checking in with yourself. As you sit there and start to settle in, your needs will come to the fore because you have made the space and time. You have made yourself available to yourself. Just engaging with yourself in this way is a mini-meditation.

As you relax a little, you might notice that you are tired. As you know, when you are working, you can be so focused on what needs to be done that you don't feel your body or your tiredness; you override those sensations. When you are "getting in," that's the time to give over, let yourself melt, let your body shift from working to resting. This tendering to yourself is the same whether you are going to meditate for a minute or twenty minutes. You may long to get on to something more "profound," but all these background sensations are the first order of business.

You may feel your skin, your muscles, your nerves vibrating. You may be aware of unfinished business in the outer and inner worlds. This is what I mean by attending to needs. Attention is drawn to your own needs. You might think you are tired, and become aware of your nerves buzzing and think you are anxious, only to discover that you are excited. As you pay attention, the sensations will tend to change.

Take a welcoming attitude toward thoughts, even if you start thinking of your to-do list. Bless your brain as if it were a cat purring.

After all, a thought is just a tiny electrical event in your neural circuitry, a millionth of a volt. Thoughts are not something to care much about.

The attitude is: *I welcome all of who I am into this space.*

It is this attitude that creates the inner sanctuary. A meditation technique is a way of finding sanctuary within yourself. Within this inner sanctuary, you can think and feel anything without fear of repercussion. You can let your hair down. Nothing counts—you are just letting your mind run wild. Your inner sanctuary is a separate state, in which you do not act on thoughts or edit them but merely witness them. If you like, you can think of it as a confessional or a therapist's couch. Nothing goes beyond these walls. This is so you can let the energies of life flow freely. From the time you begin meditating to the time you end, it's a duty-free shopping zone, a free-fire zone.

3. FEEL THE CALL TO MEDITATE

As attention settles into feeling your needs, over a period of seconds or minutes a sense of wanting to close the eyes will most likely emerge. The body wants to give over, to surrender to meditation in order to fulfill its needs to rest and renew itself. Thus, there is no sense of trying to "push" yourself into meditation or make yourself want to close the eyes. This is a very important moment, because you do not want the habit of pushing to intrude into your meditation even a little, even for a second. You are available to meditate, that is all.

The way you work this is: you sit there, aware of yourself, available, until your eyes close of their own accord. If they don't close, fine: you do an eyes-open meditation.

When the eyes eventually close, you do not do anything special. Just sit there and continue to be aware of your bodily sensations. If you have been working or playing, you will probably be aware of a peacefulness coming over you, a sense of relief and pleasure at being able to sit. If you have just awakened in the morning, you may be aware of feeling foggy and sleepy, and over time find yourself waking up. What you experience in these first few seconds will tend to be very different in the morning and in the evening.

4. MATCH RHYTHMS WITH YOURSELF

After a while of just sitting there, begin to notice the speed and impetus of your thoughts and feelings. Parts of you may feel hurried and have an urgent sense that things need to be done *now*. Other parts may be craving a vacation and want to drop out. Images, snatches of conversations, bodily feelings will come and go in a kind of rhythm. Your task here is to accommodate yourself to this rhythm. This only takes a second, but it is an essential second. Your intention should be to match rhythms with yourself. It is as if you are joining a dance, the dance of nerves and the dance of life. It is like walking into a nightclub where music is playing. You let yourself be moved by the rhythms. Every time you walk into the club, a different band will be playing, or the same band will be playing a different song.

Then, as you become one with the rhythms of your inner life, you can play with them. You can add your own, speed the band up or slow it down. When you take a conscious breath, your entire body will change its syncopation.

Matching rhythms with yourself means that sometimes you will fall through all these stages in the space of one breath, and on other occasions you might stay in just one throughout your meditation. You might notice a background sensation come up to be felt, and just attending to it might take up your entire meditation time.

Sometimes you might find that you don't even feel like closing your eyes to meditate. You might feel like going to a karaoke bar and singing your heart out. Give yourself that freedom.

5. INCLUDE AN OPENING RITUAL AND STATEMENT OF INTENTION

A ritual is some movement or thought you put forth that says "I am an individual being and I recognize that I am part of a vast universe." There are an infinite number of ways to face life and say this. You could look at a photo of the Earth from space, or a Hubbell photograph of galaxies being born, or you could think of babies, or you could pray to the Infinite. Or if it's sunny, you could go outside and soak up rays for a few minutes. I often watch the sunrise for a few minutes; then when I go inside to meditate, it is as if my being is filled with light.

You can make up your own rituals as you go. I know a woman who says, "Thank you, Lord of Life, for the gift of this day," at the beginning of every meditation. As she is saying this, her hands rise from her lap in a natural gesture of openness and thanks. This is just something she did spontaneously one day when we were working together, and she has kept on doing it. It is so natural for her and so beautiful. It makes my hair stand on end to be around her when she does this.

Other people I know say the Lord's Prayer, or read a Rumi poem, or sing a Gregorian chant in Latin. Once in Vancouver when I asked a student what prayer she felt like saying, she started saying "Hail Mary, full of grace" and the room was filled with an incredible peacefulness.

Some people will have a prayer in them that longs to come out, and others will have to go on a journey to discover it. I was raised in a religion-free family—we went surfing on Sundays—so religion was all fresh discovery to me. In 1970 when I was training to be a meditation teacher, I would meditate for forty-five minutes eight or nine times a day, with a set of yoga asanas at the beginning, after each meditation, and at the end. My yoga teacher used to say this prayer at the beginning of every set of asanas:

> *In Thy Presence, O Lord, filled with Thy Grace,*
> *I am starting yoga asanas.*
> *Grant me good health, energy, and efficiency in life.*
> *I feel Thy Grace, Thy Divine Presence.*

This little prayer, taking twenty seconds to say or think, became my favorite part of the cycle. It was the first time I had ever prayed. The sensation of doing the prayer became electric, and I would linger in the "good health, energy" part for a few extra seconds and really feel it. Even now, thinking it, I am delighted. It's as simple as a dog looking at you and wagging its tail.

If ritual is not delightful to you, then why do it? The feeling

◎ Variations

Some people like to do the same ritual every time they meditate and other people like to do something different each time. It's very individual. You might prefer one way for months or years and then change to the other.

Laughter may be your ritual. Laughter shatters the grip of small thinking and invites us into a grander scheme of things.

underneath all prayer is longing and desiring, and that is your real prayer. Being with your sense of need, longing, wonder, awe at the universe, or gratitude to be alive is your prayer. If you like to think in terms of biology, you can regard your longing for meditation as a tropism. You are turning toward meditation to satisfy a need as naturally as plants turn toward the sun.

You can keep an open and fresh attitude toward opening rituals. Meditation is ultimately the love relationship between your body and the solar system. Every breath you breathe is a cooperative action between the sun, the algae in the ocean, the forests of the world, your lungs and heart, and the muscles around your ribs. That's just a scientific fact. So whether you know it or not, every breath is an unconscious prayer. The purpose of ritually recognizing this is to free yourself from a sense of isolation. Meditation is simply paying attention to the pulse of this dance moment by moment.

NOTE: The time you spend on "getting in" to meditation is necessary, because it is not your personal will that makes meditation happen. Meditation is an activity of your total being, and you cooperate with it. Your contribution is to create conditions under which it can happen—you are inviting meditation to happen by the way you pay attention. When you take this approach, not only is meditation easy, it is effortless.

You are creating conditions under which your deepest desires can come to the surface to be attended to, and it is your movement toward fulfillment in life that drives the meditation. Meditation is not a discipline imposed from above; it comes up from the ground.

Take your time getting to know each of the stages and feeling each one throughout your body. Once you have done this, each stage can happen with a thought, or you may linger in one or more of them. It will be different every time you meditate.

If you neglect any of these stages, your meditation and your development will suffer. In my work, I have met and spoken with thousands of meditators with many years of experience, and quite a few of them have missed these simple stages. Thus, meditation still feels like an imposition to them, even after years, and they still don't know what effortlessness is.

Three Ways to Begin

The following pages contain three very different exercises. Before going farther, ask yourself what you want to do right now. Say you have fifteen minutes. Do you want to find out more about yourself by exploring your tastes and preferences? Do you want to explore your senses? Or do you want to rest and do nothing?

1. If you want to do nothing, do the Do Nothing technique.
2. If you want to get into your body, do the Salute to the Senses. Saluting one sense a day is plenty.
3. If you want to explore your individual taste, do a Feeling at Home exercise.

Just pick whichever one strikes you right now. They are all easy, and at some point you will want to do all of them.

Meditation is not just a set of techniques. It is your relationship with yourself, and the techniques emerge from that relationship. If you pay attention to your relationship with breath, or with sound, or with sensation or light, you yourself can invent any number of meditation practices.

Remember, there is no "end goal" of meditation. It is a tool to help you enhance your appreciation for the gift of life.

The methods in this book are presented as a way for you to get your feet wet. Once you are exploring, though, you will receive feedback from your inner and outer life. I encourage you to change the techniques and make them your own as you learn them. Your instinctive wisdom will guide you. People can be harmed by relying too much on external authority. Develop the habit of checking in with yourself about each technique, about what you want to do and how long you want to do it. This will activate your instinctive self-knowing. The habits you start with will tend to persist.

Do not expect anything in particular to happen at any given moment when you are meditating. It is enough just to sit and be relatively restful.

> **Tip:** *Always give yourself permission to say no and not meditate right now. Maybe tomorrow you will find yourself different. Do not feel that you need to impose meditation on yourself. If you can say no today, you can also say yes.*

Beginners often say:

- It's a relief just to sit still.
- The air has a silky texture in my throat.
- The movement of the breath is soothing.
- I like the rhythm.
- Is this really meditation? I feel like I am just sitting here being myself.
- I like the feeling of drawing the breath in really deep.
- I like the little pause at the end, before you exhale.
- As I am sitting here, I feel perfectly at home in myself.
- I can feel myself letting go of fatigue and getting charged up.
- I have the feeling I'm going to have a good day after this meditation.
- Walking around the block after meditating, I feel so relaxed in my body, every movement is a pleasure. I am glad just to be alive.
- I never appreciated how beautiful silence is before; it's almost musical.

I. THE DO NOTHING TECHNIQUE

TIME: 3 minutes to 5 minutes.
POSTURE: Lying down or sitting.
WHEN: Anytime.

Sit or lie down and just allow your mind to do its thing. Your aim is to tolerate being there without trying to control anything. If you can do this, congratulate yourself. Take yourself to lunch. Your path in meditation is going to be pretty simple.

Let your attention go anywhere it wants. You can think about sex, your to-do lists, movies, nothing, everything.

Notice where your mind goes. The only thing that makes this seem even vaguely like a meditation is that you have given yourself a time frame of three to five minutes.

This exercise helps you overcome technique-itis, which is the notion that there is something to be afraid of or that the human mind somehow has to be controlled even when you are resting. Technique-itis, left untreated, is mildly contagious and tends to last for ten to fifteen years, or until you give up on meditation forever.

To develop an immunity to technique-itis, simply Do Nothing and tolerate whatever your body and mind do. You want to be in the same state you're in when you are about to fall asleep. The mind is just drifting. You need to find out if you can take whatever happens when you release control.

You will learn to experience your natural state, without *doing* anything to it. Many people are slightly ashamed of their unvarnished selves and look for "techniques" to "improve" themselves. Years later, they are still doing gadgetry to themselves, and often nothing has changed.

Variation No. 1

Close your eyes and pretend you are taking a nap—only you don't have to fall asleep. This is a conscious nap. You can make things very cozy. You can build a fire in the fireplace, wrap yourself in a blanket, and just look at the fire. Or you can lie down. If you fall asleep and have a real nap, no problem. Just do the exercise when you wake up.

How does doing this exercise differ from being a couch potato? You are intentionally doing nothing. You do not even have to approach meditation as a technique, although you may if you wish. Notice what your attitudes are, and do not defend yourself against anything. Whether you are reverent, irreverent, bored, happy, tired, or excited, welcome it all. You cannot fail.

Variation No. 2

Pray and then meditate. You could say your favorite prayers to create an atmosphere of safety, and then let go and Do Nothing.

Tips: *It's okay if you can't tolerate doing nothing, but that is the place from which you start.*

If you have a lot of noise in your head while Doing Nothing, you may find yourself wanting to take action in some form—clean up your room or clean up your act. All that "noise" or mental rehearsal is not a problem and is not to be resisted. Your brain needs to do it.

If you find yourself afraid of keeping yourself company, and a certain percentage of people do, then make sure you proceed at your own pace. You could begin by meditating only in places where you feel really safe, whether that is in your room, in a church or temple, at the beach, or in a theater between movies.

Problem: If you have a sleep debt, doing nothing will probably put you to sleep.

Solution: Most people have at least a few hours of sleep debt. Just take naps instead of meditating, and maybe go to bed half an hour earlier for a few weeks. If you take care of it, you will feel much better, and you won't fall asleep when you are meditating. As a bonus, you might not get that cold that's going around, because you won't be so run-down. You can't learn to meditate if you are fighting sleep.

2. SALUTE TO THE SENSES

TIME: 3 minutes to 5 minutes for each sense.
POSTURE: Standing, walking, lying down, or sitting.
WHEN: Anytime except when operating heavy machinery.

Let's take a tour of some of the commonly known human senses. All of them are employed in the various meditation techniques of the world, by themselves and in combination.

Attention and mindfulness happen through the senses. When you are aware of thinking, it is through internal sensing: you see a mental image in your "mind's eye"; you hear a thought or you feel one. You can even call up thought-smells.

The meditations in this section touch on all the senses, not just seeing and hearing and taste and touch and smell, but also balance and movement. Take the time to explore these brief sensory salutations, at your own pace. You could take a year or you could take a month to go through them. If you are on vacation, you could do them in a couple of days. But the real effects will show up over the long run, over the months and years.

The first few times you do one of these exercises, it may take many minutes to engage fully with one of the senses and experience its range. Over time, however, simply thinking of one of the senses for a moment will awaken it. Tuning into each of your senses every day will enrich your life in subtle and wonderful ways.

> **Tip:** Some people run into tremendous guilt when Doing Nothing. The exercise directly challenges their work ethic—and their fear of nothingness. Many of those people have been unable to work through their guilt. It is simple, though: if you feel bad doing nothing, just keep coming back and facing the feeling directly, and eventually you will win. The problem with not clearing out this feeling is that doing nothing is part of resting. Such people tend to work to exhaustion and then drop. Or they have to drink or smoke to get into rest. Or have sex as an escape rather than just for fun or love. Lots of people who seem to be happily meditating are tying themselves up in rules out of fear of doing nothing. They have all kinds of invisible rules and regulations.

The more you let your senses open up and rejoice in meditation, the better. When you pay attention to a sense, it comes alive. If you do so consistently, the brain literally creates more neural pathways to appreciate that sense.

The brain rewires itself daily to be better at what we are paying attention to. When you exercise a sense, the brain makes more neural connections for that sensory pathway. When you connect that sense with other senses, the brain makes connective pathways to coordinate perceptions. This is one of the things that makes meditation so much fun: you progressively have richer experiences of your body and your world as you move through your daily life.

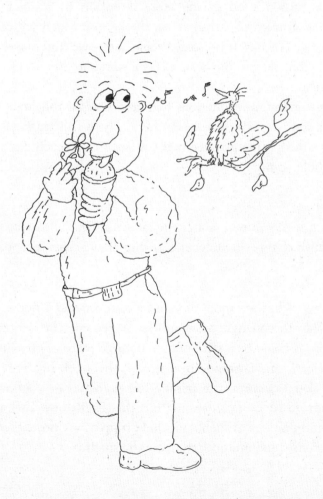

As you read through the following paragraphs, linger a bit and evoke your senses by calling up your favorite ways of experiencing. Take an attitude of playful idleness when exploring the senses, at least the first couple of times you explore each sense. Play and childlike curiosity engage your instincts in a healthy way and help you establish an easy familiarity with your senses. In an informal approach to meditation, this is the way to go.

Doing the Salute to the Senses is very simple. After all, these are the senses you use all the time to know where you are in the world and how you are doing. The exercises below are ways of celebrating every-day sensuous perceptions. You will be choosing a sense—hearing, or touch, or vision—and paying close attention to it. Not much is required to awaken the senses; even the lightest touch suffices to start the process. The payoff is usually immediate—we find ourselves just a little bit more alert to the beauty of the world around us. Go for those tiny changes.

Grab some mini-meditations here and there throughout your day. Two minutes here, thirty seconds there. These will teach you how to develop a meditation practice that you want to do each day. And that is the whole point.

Smell

How it works: Smell is a chemical sense that allows us to detect the electric charge on molecules as they flow across receptors in the nose.

Explore: What are some of your favorite smells? Choose one that is available to you right now and let it become the center of your attention. It could be a stick of cinnamon, a piece of chewing gum, a leaf, a cigar, a rose, brandy in a snifter, the smell of the leather on your pocket organizer, the perfume or cologne on your wrist. You could just go sit in a garden and breathe. Right now I thought of a peach, and one was available so I held it up to my nose, breathing in and out for several minutes, studying the smell.

Salute to Smell

1. *Select something with a smell you want to enjoy. If possible, hold the object in your hand. It could be a piece of orange, a flower, a bottle of perfume, chocolate, wine, a cigar, anything. Try to have fresh air, or clean air, where you are meditating.*

2. *Sit in a comfortable place.*

3. *Place the item near your nose and breathe in its scent.*

4. *Notice where in your nose the sense of smell seems to come from.*

5. *Be aware of changes in the experience of smell as you become saturated with the odor.*

6. *Be alert to sensations coming from your entire body as you breathe the smell in and out. Depending on your mood and the nature of the smell, you might have tingling or melting sensations on your skin or in your belly, genitals, heart area, or legs. The smell might be evocative of emotions. Let those emotions move through you, and attend to them as long as you like; then return to the sense of smell. If the emotions come back and are strong, attend to the places in your body with physical sensations that correlate to the emotion. If, for example, a perfume reminds you of a time or place you once wore it, and you have a longing about that, is the longing in your heart area? Is it in your gut, your belly? Is it in your entire upper torso?*

7. *After several minutes, move the item away, so that there is only the barest hint of its smell.*

8. *After several more minutes, move the item farther away, so that no discernible hint of it remains, only the possibility that a molecule or two of it will reach your nose.*
   Yet, stay alert in your nose to the possibility of smell, and continue being aware of breathing, being alert to the presence of nothing in the air. You are alert, you are mindful in the nose, but there is nothing there except pure air. This exercise is really about waking up to smell.

Over time, this meditation will increase your alertness to smells, even the smell of pure, clean air. You can be sitting under a tree, or on your sofa, and draw in a breath of fresh air and enjoy air. You can draw energy out of air. You can draw calmness out of air. You can draw any quality you crave out of the air. If you cultivate your sense of smell, you will also cultivate your ability to be alert to the whole process of breathing, and your meditations will be that much more enjoyable.

Taste

How it works: Taste is a chemical sense that detects the ions and molecules touching your tongue.

There is much more to it, of course. Taste is inextricably linked with many other senses on and in the tongue: the sense of temperature and texture, the movement sensors in the tongue, and the muscularity of chewing. When we eat something and savor the taste of it, even the way it looked before we put it in our mouth is part of the experience. The sound of the crunch as we chew is part of the whole delight. Let all these other impressions come and go as you taste, but let taste be the center of your focus.

Explore: What are some of your favorite tastes? I just ate some sushi, and the taste of the ginger and horseradish is lingering in my mouth. Is there anything around that you would like to taste? Take a little bite of it.

Salute to Taste

After air, water is our most essential need. Water has a taste when we are thirsty—it tastes good. Even distilled water tastes good. (You could also use fruit juice or wine for this exercise.)

1. *Taste a sip of water. Sample it little by little. Do not completely satisfy your thirst until later.*

2. *Notice how the water affects the sensations in your mouth. Where are you experiencing taste? How does your tongue, the roof of your mouth, the back of your throat welcome the water? Have you ever noticed this before?*

3. *Scan your body for sensations that go with drinking water. What happens in your belly? How does your attitude change as you sip?*

4. *After a couple of minutes, gulp as much of the water as you like. Gulp attentively if you can. Notice the sensations in the belly.*

Check out your body for the subtle, pleasurable sensations of being satisfied.

When you have gotten used to this technique, you may find that anytime you drink water you can turn on your sense of taste and really enjoy. It may take only two seconds, but you have enjoyed a simple, everyday experience.

If you like, you could use a sip of water at the beginning of a meal to key you in to enhanced taste. You may find that this helps you eat only as much as you need, and enjoy it more, without getting into control issues with food. This is one of the purposes of having wine with meals. There is so much to smell in a glass of wine, and every sip has such a complex taste, that the whole body is prepared for sensual enjoyment of food.

Your experience may be different each time you do this exercise. It will depend on your state of relaxation, how hydrated you are, the outside temperature and humidity, your emotional state, where you are, and the particular water you are tasting. Emotions may come up that relate to times when you were really thirsty. Pictures may come into your head. Be with the emotions and pictures, and when they fade away, return to the sense of taste. Every time your mind wanders, it is clearing out cobwebs and bringing the richness of memory to the present moment.

Sight

How it works: Special cells in your retina contain molecules that respond to light waves pulsing in the range of about four hundred trillion to eight hundred trillion times a second. Your brain translates this information into the experience of color, texture, depth, shape, and motion. A great deal of the brain is devoted to visual processing.

Explore: Let your gaze wander around the room or area you are in right now. Notice how effortlessly the eyes move. Release the eyes from any control and just let them move wherever they want.

Salute to Sight

1. *Let your eyes move around and then alight on some color that calls you. Allow your eyes to rest on the color. The eyes may move, but they can also feel at ease. Ask yourself, what colors or sights do I crave right now? Would you like to be in Tahiti, looking out over the ocean? In a forest or in the mountains? Looking at the body of your lover? Let images stream though your mind's eye if you like.*

There is sometimes a sensation of being touched by light, when the light is right and the mood is right. Be alert for subtle sensations in the eyes as you notice your reaction to color.

The eyes can feel extraordinarily restful while we are seeing. Sometimes we reach out to grab the world with our eyes, but we can also experience being receptive to color—which is the case in reality. Although the eyes move, it is the electromagnetic spectrum entering the eyes that makes the molecules excited.

2. *Now let your eyes move around and alight on some texture of the visual world. Texture is the surface of the objects you are seeing. Choose a texture that appeals to you and be aware of it for half a minute.*

3. *Do the same with the depth of field. Notice that you can tell how much empty space is between you and all the objects you see. Notice the empty space, the air between you and the objects you are seeing.*

4. *Become aware of your peripheral vision. Rest the eyes on some spot in front of you, and with the peripheral vision, see to the left and right, above and below.*

5. *Notice the element of shape in the objects you are seeing. And if the objects are moving or static, how they sit in space.*

Just touch on these items for half a minute or so. Your aim is simply to notice some of the range and quality of vision, and to stay there for a few seconds.

Hearing

How it works: Inside each ear is a resonant chamber with tens of thousands of tiny hairs of different lengths. Each hair vibrates to a different frequency of sound waves, setting off nerve cells. Your brain takes the impulses coming from these cells and sends the data swirling around intricate neural circuitry. This gives you the experience of tone, resonance, amplitude, direction, and many other wonderful qualities. The filtering mechanism lets you pick one conversation out of many at a party.

Explore: Is there a simple sound that you would like to hear? Or would you prefer silence? Give yourself a moment to wonder what quality or intensity of sound or silence you would like to experience.

Salute to Hearing

1. *Sit in a place where there is a sound you like, perhaps the sound of a fountain or a bird. Or sit where you are and listen to the sound of life around you, whether it is distant traffic, kids playing in a yard, the television in the next room, or someone walking back and forth above you.*

2. *After listening with the eyes open for a minute or two, close the eyes and continue listening. Let yourself keep track of what is going on, and notice the three-dimensionality of sound. If you have two functional ears, you can locate noises in all directions, including up and down.*

3. *Begin to pay attention to the relative quiet between sounds—if there is any. If not, then notice the space between you and the source of the sounds. You can usually tell, by listening, how far away the source of the sound is.*

4. *Put your attention in the ears themselves and be awake there, listening and feeling. This will be easier if the sounds around you are not too loud.*

Touch

How it works: In the skin are many sensors for detecting touch, pressure, heat, and pain, and each of these has its own specialized nerve terminals. Just within touch itself, there are nerves for sensing the light contact that moves the hairs, a touch on the skin surface itself, and a strong touch. The skin has sensors both near the surface and deeper in the tissue.

Explore: Check in with your body right now and ask yourself, what touch do I want? Touch anything with eyes closed and experience the sensations in your fingertips and palms, as if touching for the first time. Touch your skull very lightly and lovingly; let your hands and the skin of your scalp be awake to each other.

Variation

Touch different textures, such as fur, silk, velvet, wool, carpet, wood, and glass. Touch different areas of your skin. Have someone touch you all over very lightly. Have someone breathe on your skin. Experiment with different pressures, light and strong, fast and slow. In terms of touch, meditation sometimes feels like the most delicate foreplay imaginable.

Salute to Touch

1. *Starting at the top of the head, with an extremely light touch, move down the midline of the body. Move extremely slowly. Use one hand, perhaps the middle finger. Go as far down as you feel comfortable.*

   Experiment by moving your hand or finger away from the body, then back in slowly. Notice the point at which you can tell that your finger is about to touch.

2. *Notice which areas of the body crave to be touched lightly. Explore the forehead, the eyelids, the lips, the hollow of the throat, the area between the breasts, the belly, and if you are so inclined, areas around the genitals.*

3. *Hold the hands in front of the chest, palms inward, and move them in and out a few inches as you breathe. On the inbreath, let the hands come all the way in and lightly touch the chest. On the outbreath, move them slightly out.*

Each area of the body has its own relationship with touch and preference for kinds of touch. The lips, hands, and genitals have lots of nerve endings.

Kinesthesia

How it works: There are nerves in the muscles to detect stretch and tension, and there are nerves in the joints to detect position. You can notice these whenever you are sitting or lying down and breathing, or when you are walking, running, swimming, dancing, making love, or doing yoga.

Explore: Consider the many movements you do every day, from the time you get out of bed in the morning to the time you go to sleep at night. Which movements do you love in particular? Which ones do you pay attention to? Which ones would you miss terribly if you were no longer able to do them?

Salute to Movement Sensing

1. *Let one or both of your hands move as if you were gesturing in a conversation. But let the movement be very slow. Now close your eyes and continue, noticing not only the sensations in your arms and hands, but those all over your body.*

2. *Let the movements gradually become slower and slower until you are moving so slowly that even you can't tell if you are moving or not.*

3. *Stand with the eyes closed and swing your arms from side to side. Move with vigor and enthusiasm and then slow down gradually. Notice how you detect movement. Notice how it makes you feel, how it changes your mood.*

4. *Still standing there with eyes closed, know where your joints are in space. You can tell instantly. Simply notice that you know where your joints and limbs are.*

Balance

How it works: Near the inner ears are semicircular canals (vestibules) filled with fluid. Whenever the fluid moves, it causes movement in tiny hairs lining the canal, and sensors detect this. The brain interprets this information as the relationship with gravity, the mysterious attraction that matter has for matter. Balance, also called the vestibular sense, alerts your brain continually to the relationship of the body to the center of the Earth.

Explore: Whenever you are moving, accelerating, standing, sitting, or lying down, you are enjoying the sense of balance. But the vestibular sense works so seamlessly and cooperates so beautifully with vision and kinesthesia that we rarely experience it in itself. Anytime you lean over, you can feel gravity attracting you.

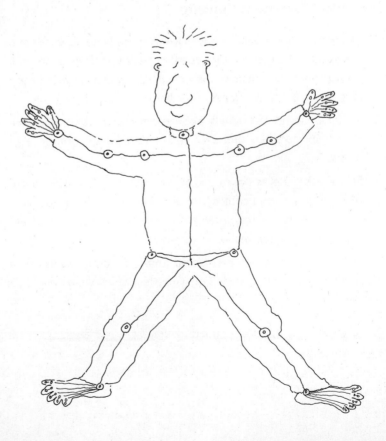

Salute to Balance

1. *Sitting with eyes closed, tilt your head very slightly one way and then the other: left, then right. Notice the sense that informs you when your head is at the centerline. Let your movements be tiny, a fraction of an inch.*

2. *After you get used to the small head movements, explore doing tiny spiral or circular motions around where the center is, around where perfect vertical is.*

3. *There is an exquisite feeling right at the vertical. You can sense this if you are moving slowly enough. Continue to play with being off-center, then "falling upwards" toward center. When you get used to this sense of vertical, through playing around with being slightly off-balance, there comes a sense of great pleasure in being upright.*

Your Relationship with the Senses

All the senses are used in meditation. Stay with any of these sensuous modalities for a minute or so to let yourself be reminded of what's real. Each sense is both external—as in hearing a sound—and internal, as in hearing the thought of the sound or hearing yourself think. Anyone with the sense of hearing can call up at will a remembered sound, and similarly people can call up an image or a feeling. Each sense reaches into the outer world and into the inner world.

The senses constantly blend and interact with one another, and a single sense rarely operates in isolation. When you are eating, you see the food, smell it, taste it, feel the motion as you bite into it, and feel it move around in your mouth before swallowing it. Then you feel satisfied, which is yet another sensation. When you are walking, you look around, smell the air, hear cars and people on all sides of you, feel the motion in your legs, and feel hot or cold. When you are in a passionate embrace, there is something for every sense to enjoy. When you are listening to music, you will find that you are processing not only auditory

NOTE: If one of your senses is impaired, you can still salute it. You can even salute its absence! Whenever we are deprived of one sense, the others become more sensitive to compensate. So if any of your senses are impaired, be creative in inventing and adapting. I have always envied people who speak ASL (American Sign Language) and other sign languages, because they are so beautiful to watch. Someday I want to meet a meditation teacher who is deaf and has explored the use of sign language in meditation.

signals but also kinesthetic information from all over your body. And no matter what you are doing, sitting still or moving, your sense of balance is always there informing you.

In meditation you use the same senses that you use when you are enjoying yourself. So the more intimate you become with the senses, the better. As you salute each of the senses, you give it permission to interact with the others in new ways.

Take the time to make a sensuous inventory. What are your dominant senses? Which ones are the least developed? Be willing to refresh your relationship with each of the sensory pathways. Each connects you to the outer world and the inner world in a different way, and the variations and combinations are infinite.

Although it may seem extremely simple, saluting the senses is a profound exercise. Even a few minutes a day of doing this will, over time, change your experience of life in interesting and useful ways.

If you are a beginner at meditation, then you have a great advantage. You have not learned to split "the spiritual" from common, everyday sensuous perception. And if you do not ever split yourself in this way, then you will not have to quit meditating someday in order to recover from the split and reunify yourself.

The more alert you are to all the senses, the richer your meditations will be, the more textured your sense of your inner world. Even thinking is a sensory experience; when we are thinking, we see inner pictures, we move them around and look at them from different angles, we listen to our internal dialogues, and we feel different body sensations with each of the scenarios we create.

Meditators often get into a rut with their senses, using the same ones in the same way every day. When asked to "Scan your body" or "Pay attention to breath," people will use whatever senses they are accustomed to working with. But even in a simple experience of breath, there is sound, movement, touch, balance, and perhaps smell. The more senses you enjoy in meditation, the richer your experience will be. It only takes a minute to orbit through all the senses and give them permission to play. When you get intimate with a sense, you are saying to it, "Talk to me, tell me your story. What do you want?" The senses always answer, each in its unique way.

After meditation, go and use your senses.

All Senses Meditation

TIME: 5 minutes to 10 minutes.

POSTURE: Sitting is preferable. You can also experiment with lying
  down or standing.

WHEN: Anytime.

All Senses Meditation

This exercise lets you play with orbiting through your senses and observing something in each.

1. *Sit or stand anywhere you like and let yourself "get in" for a minute. Do any settling-down movements that you want. Stretch or yawn. Then notice the ebb and flow of your breathing.*

2. *Begin to speak softly, saying "Now I am aware of seeing . . ." Continue by saying whatever comes to mind that is visual, whether it is in the outer world or a mental image. The sentence can be said very slowly. Go on like this for a minute or so, just speaking the sentence "Now I am aware of seeing . . ."*

3. *When you get to the word seeing, say whatever image your mind or eyes are on at that exact moment. As in "I am aware of seeing the rain."*

4. *Switch to another sensory mode, "Now I am aware of smelling . . . ," and say whatever you are smelling.*

5. *Continue this way, starting each sentence with "Now I am aware . . ." and then choosing another sense. Improvise off your immediate perceptions.*

NOTE: In the All Senses meditation, what happens is that your primary perceptions, unsocialized, get a chance to come out without editing. This trains you to let yourself be surprised by perception, to let new and fresh perceptions emerge.

The exercise also allows you to practice giving speech freely to your immediate perceptions. Since childhood, you may not have had a chance to speak without editing first.

NOTE: In the All Senses meditation, you may move through the senses in any order you wish:

> *Now I am aware of seeing . . .*
> *Now I am aware of smelling . . .*
> *Now I am aware of hearing . . .*
> *Now I am aware of tasting . . .*
> *Now I am aware of touching . . .*
> *Now I am aware of moving . . .*
> *Now I am aware of balance . . .*

3. FEELING AT HOME EXERCISE

TIME: 5 minutes to 10 minutes.
POSTURE: Sitting or lying down.
WHEN: Anytime you feel like it.

To begin the Feeling at Home exercise for meditation, ask yourself, when have I felt really at home? Really at home in myself? Call up an experience and breathe with it for a few minutes. That's all. The following paragraphs are a meditation induction, meant to be read slowly. They're repetitive because the process is one of calling forth an experience, breathing with it, then letting it go and shifting to a different aspect of the experience and breathing with that.

Set your mind free to wander over your life experience and recall instances when you have felt very, very comfortable. They could have occurred anywhere, anytime, under any conditions.

If you like, get some paper and jot down all the times you can think of when you felt at home, in yourself, in your body, in the world, or in your heart. Each note can be a brief reminder, a couple of words. Then select one at a time and go into it deeply and let it teach you. Soak in it with all your senses.

As each impression and each aspect of the experience comes to mind, let it also come to your senses and your body. Let yourself see with your mind's eye what you saw, feel what you felt, hear what you heard, smell what you smelled, taste what you tasted.

If one of your memories of being at home is standing on the shore, there is the smell of the salt air, the sound of the surf, wind, and seagulls, the wetness of the spray on your face, the brilliance of the sun or the gray of the clouds, and the blue rolling motion of the ocean. Immerse yourself in each of these; let yourself rejoice in each sense.

Perhaps you recall a time when you walked for hours in the mountains and then rested under a tree overlooking a meadow. Let yourself recall that moment in rich sensory detail. You may have been aware of the buzz of fatigue in your muscles, a feeling of expansion in your heart as you looked out at the meadow nestled in the mountains, the ease with which your eyes took it all in, the beauty of sunlight shimmering on a stream, the quiet sound of brush rustling in the breeze.

As the images and memories come, breathe with them. Enter the image, see the scene, breathe with the feeling you had in your body. When you do this, the feelings come into the present. You are, in the present moment, meditating on the feeling of "being at home."

When you are feeling at home, how do your eyes work?
When you are at home, how do you experience sound?
How does your skin feel?

Allow the memory to infuse you, take you over, teach you, bless you. Bless the memory in turn, and give thanks to life for the gift of being at home.

In so doing, you are giving your body a chance to learn from the condition of being at home. You are learning from your own spontaneous experiences. You are learning how your senses operate when you are at ease, at home in yourself.

Recalling an experience brings up the way your brain and sensory

Tip: *If you are tired or under stress, do not do the Feeling at Home exercise unless you seem to fall into it. Instead, find one of the breathing practices to enjoy. Someday soon, when you have more energy for it, come back and explore being at home.*

nervous system and breath function when you are in that experience. When you associate that with your breathing now, today, it alerts your brain to let meditation be just as friendly and inviting.

Keep returning to this exercise over and over when you have quiet time. If you like to write, you could keep a journal about your experiences. The primary task is to let your senses, all of them, be refreshed by the process of recollection. You will find that the process gets faster. Soon, the positive qualities you love about life will be at your fingertips to call upon whenever you need to. You may find, too, that your memory improves.

Do this exercise for a few minutes, and if it is going really well, continue it for as long as you like. Let your experience be leisurely.

Each time you do the exercise you may recall different experiences: holding your baby, sailing, dancing all night, sleeping under the stars while camping, a long and wonderful conversation with a friend, a vacation cruise, the day you graduated from a school, riding a horse. It will teach you about the way your senses operate when you are having vivid, life-affirming experiences.

Surprisingly, many people who learn meditation never learn to be at home in the practice. They always feel they are doing a technique coming from outside the self, and the authority for how to do the technique resides in India or Tibet or Japan.

Your meditation practice for the first month could be simply remembering times that you've felt at home in the world, spending five minutes or so a day in this way. If you think that sounds too simple, try it!

Variations

You can also do the Feeling at Home exercise with experiences such as feeling intensely alive, being extremely alert, being flooded with gratitude, and experiencing love. Each of these will teach you something different about your natural gateways into heightened attention. Cultivating your attention in this way will be a great gift to your life and to your path in meditation.

The secret is so simple that it is easy to overlook. When you bring up a memory and breathe with it in the present moment, your entire nervous system is alerted to that way of functioning and, if it is appropriate, will make use of those sensory pathways.

In private instruction, I spend much of the time listening as people tell me about their experiences of being at home, being in love, being in gratitude to be alive. As they access the memories, they go into meditation spontaneously, in their own natural way. Then I interview them while they are meditating and have them teach me about their individual paths.

You can do this on your own. It may take a little longer because no one but you is there holding the space for you. But you can do it. If tears come, let them come. If regret comes, let it come. You are not doing anything unnatural to yourself; you are simply engaging in an honest process of reflecting on and learning from your experiences.

Over time, you may find that once you open the gate, these experiences come of their own accord, each seeking to give you its gift. Accept the gift.

This exercise is not just an indulgence. Doing it for even a few seconds a day gives the body a sense of remembered wellness. This strengthens the immune system, reminds you of what life is all about, and makes you emotionally more resilient and self-sufficient.

Each of these spontaneous experiences is your teacher. Your task is to savor these experiences periodically and let them instruct you. It is a body-based teaching: your nerves practice doing what is involved in the experience as you remember. This gives your body permission to feel the same way when you are meditating. And ultimately, you will meditate every day if you feel safe doing so. You will learn to function in a state of relaxation, without pushing your panic button all the time, if you feel safe to do so. You will learn to move through your world with your senses wide-open. The Feeling at Home exercise will not interfere in any way with your ability to panic if you really need to, or if the emergency response is needed. This exercise just clears the roadway, making you better able to feel at home in the world if it is appropriate to do so.

Getting Out

Always give yourself leisure time at the end of a meditation session. Allow about three minutes. This "getting out" time is as important as the meditation itself; it is your segue into action. And the whole point of meditation is to carry the relaxed attentiveness into action.

Pause Now and
Take a Deep Breath

1. You become aware that you are going to end the meditation soon. You could call it an intention—you are just aware for a split second that you are going to get up soon. The body will immediately shift from healing mode into a kind of neutral gear.

2. You do nothing, you just coast. Thoughts can come and go, sensations come and go, you are not intending anything. Several minutes of this may seem like a really long time, a whole world of experience. You need a watch at hand to make sure you stay there.

3. Toward the end of the getting-out time, make little movements. Sigh. Then wait a few seconds. Then make a movement again. You will feel your metabolism begin to speed up.

4. Open the eyes a little, then close them again and notice your inner feelings. You will probably sigh again. Again open the eyes, a little more. Perhaps look downward and in front of you for a few seconds, because that means the eyelids do not have to open all the way.

5. Open the eyes and simply sit there for half a minute, savoring your body sensations.

CLOSING RITUALS

I recommend that people make up their own closing rituals, using hand and arm gestures. For example, slowly open the arms wide, then bring them in so the hands are over the heart. Then again open the arms, and bring the hands in to rest on the belly. Learn to appreciate a very slow movement here, slower than you've ever made before. Move at the speed you can feel. This slow movement helps the body integrate inner and outer.

For a one-minute meditation, there is no need to do any rituals for getting out. But for a ten- or twenty-minute meditation, make it a rule to spend about a minute reorienting for every five minutes you were meditating. This is something you have to impose on yourself, because spending two minutes at the end of a ten-minute meditation seems like forever. You may find yourself sitting there going vroom, vroom, revving your engines, eager to leap into action. If you have deadlines or are anxious about your performance at something, this vroom time is actually more important than the other parts of meditation. Your body is practicing staying as relaxed as possible while feeling the urgency to act and perhaps rehearsing specific actions.

If you have a limited amount of time for your whole meditation—say you have twenty minutes in all—then you work backward to see how much time you can spend with your eyes closed. Subtracting a minute or two at the beginning, and three at the end, plus a couple of minutes thrown in as a buffer, leaves you about fourteen minutes for eyes-closed meditation. It is much better to have these interlude moments for the transitions.

I once had a student who was an ER doctor, an emergency room specialist. He worked long shifts, and often nothing was happening, so he could rest in a room near the ER. On occasion, however, he would have to get up from meditation at a dead run and deal with a patient. He said that after doing this once, and being a bit shocked, his body invented an "intermediate" meditation state for when he was at the hospital, in which it kept guard with one part and let him mostly rest. He said he felt like a dog "sleeping with one eye open," except that he meditated with one eye open. When he was at home meditating, he would go much deeper because he knew he wouldn't be interrupted.

So know that you can get up out of meditation at a dead run if you should ever have to, but don't do it unless you have to.

◎ Going Deeper

The Sensuous Texture of Daily Life

There is a sensuous texture to everyday living. Awakening in the morning, you feel a certain way when you first come to consciousness. Then there is the first stretch, and you open your eyes to see what time it is. Standing in the shower you may or may not savor the water flowing on your skin. Drinking your coffee or tea, you may celebrate the taste or just mechanically consume it. As you look around at the people you love, your heart may be filled with love, or you may be too busy in your mind to really see them.

At work, sometimes the day flows as if you have inner resources backing you up, and sometimes it drags. Going to lunch, you may be happy or anxious. Coming home, there is the way you feel when you walk in the door. You may be ecstatic to be home and glad to see everyone, or you may bring the stress of work right in with you. Going to bed, there is the way you feel getting under the covers and what you think about lying there. What were your last thoughts as you went to sleep last night? Each of these moments borders on meditation and is a good path to take inward. It is up to you to allow yourself to go with the moment and permit it to deepen. To do so means you have to assess how much time you have, how safe you are, what it is you are curious about. The senses are the way into meditation and also the means you use to verify whether meditation is working for you in your life.

You can tell that meditation is working by the tiny, barely noticeable changes in the sensory quality of your day, by how you feel doing your life. The mundane is where your teacher is. Make the everyday your teacher, your guide. By noticing the feedback from your everyday life, you will be able to tell how you are doing. Other people may be able to see the changes as well. They may say, "You seem in a better mood lately."

Explore your way through the meditations in this section. There is no rule about which to do first, which not to do at all. Let your cravings and your needs guide you. Everyone has rituals for getting ready for the day; everyone has to rise and shine in some way. Paying a bit more attention while doing your everyday rituals of bathing and getting ready for the day is a good way to get into meditation. You can begin the process of building a daily meditation practice in this way, doing what you do anyway. Most of these meditations can be done in secret. No one will even know that you are doing anything special.

Life is a succession of little moments, inner and outer. We know of these moments through our many senses. The more alert we are in the senses, the more there is to notice of the texture of the world and the texture of our feelings, sensations, and thoughts. The point of meditation is to see the Earth with fresh eyes, to become a person upon whom nothing is lost. Your way will probably be different from anyone else's. Find your own way into little meditation moments such as are described on the following pages. Invent your own, using my suggestions as hints or templates.

To select any of these sensory meditations, just pick your favorites, the ones that immediately attract you. After a week or two or a month, pick one that is unfamiliar. Treat them as recipes in a cookbook. Someday you may want to try each one. The main thing you are up to is training yourself to stay with a pleasurable sensation for longer than you ordinarily would, for thirty seconds, a minute, three minutes.

Mini-Meditations Throughout the Day

WAKE UP AND SMELL THE COFFEE

TIME: Give it 15 minutes. I dare you. But you can do it in 5 minutes.
WHEN: Morning, or soon after arising.

NOTE: You may feel that somehow you are violating a taboo by paying attention to your coffee, that there is some sort of rule against actually smelling and tasting for more than a couple of seconds. No one is allowed to have this much fun with something so simple. You may find yourself becoming anxious, even if you have plenty of time to get ready for work. Anytime you break a perceived taboo, a warning buzzer goes off. Pay attention to this and don't push it too much in any one day. Simply notice the rule about not really paying attention, and come back tomorrow.

You can use sipping your morning drink as a meditation in itself, and also as a way into a longer meditation. Many successful meditators I know use commonplace rituals such as this as a gateway to meditation.

If you are doing this mini-meditation in the morning, shower first, then drink some water so you aren't thirsty.

Get a cup of your favorite warm drink—coffee, tea, herb tea—and sit somewhere comfortable where you can hold the cup and rest. Hold it under your nose and breathe in and out. This is normal savoring activity, only you stay with it longer. Keep on paying attention right through your usual limit, whether it is one second or ten.

Hold the cup in both hands and at just the right distance from your nose. You can close the eyes and give over to smell. You are breathing in and out as you smell, so enjoy the flow. Notice the sensations you have in your belly as you inhale the smell of your coffee. Be alert for sensations anywhere in your body.

Breathe in the smell for a while, then take a taste. Notice what happens in the mouth and on the tongue as you sip. Notice what happens in the entire body.

Put the cup down on a table, or lower your hands and hold the cup in your lap, and enjoy yourself.

Then raise the cup again. Make this a ritual movement, slow and gracious.

Continue this rhythm of breathing in the smell and resting for a few minutes.

Many senses besides smell and taste are involved in enjoying a cup of coffee. Sight brings you information about colors and shapes; touch informs you of the warmth of the cup and the smoothness of its surface; your motion sensors feed you sensations as you lift the cup to your lips.

> *Tip:* When we do things habitually, without paying much attention, we ignore feedback from our bodies. Many people, when they start paying attention while eating and drinking, find that they don't actually like what they're putting in their mouths. Sometimes they discover they don't like coffee, now that they are really tasting it; they like certain teas or prefer water and juice. Or they find that they are satisfied with just a sip and do not want to gulp.
>
> Be prepared to study your preferences as you start paying more attention to taste. And take the time to explore what you really love to sip in the morning, at lunch, in the afternoon, and during the evening. If it's good coffee, freshly roasted, have that. If it is herb tea or juice, have it available.

ARRIVE EARLY FOR EVERYTHING

TIME: About 3 minutes.

WHEN: At every scheduled meeting.

If you are even a little early for the events of your day, you can take a moment to breathe, feel yourself, and enjoy. It's a little luxury that meditators often overlook. One minute here and there can change the whole rhythm of a day by allowing you to catch up with yourself. This simple step will alter your life significantly, unless you are already hip to it.

I get the feeling that in the military "on time" means you arrive five minutes early, then stand around preparing yourself to walk in the door at the exact second of the appointment. At least, that's how military types I have worked with come for their meditation sessions. It doesn't matter whether they are generals, captains, or sergeants. They always seem to arrive early, loaf around outside, then knock on the door right on time. I can set my watch by them. Since they are not out of breath, it's easier for them to get into breath awareness. And they are very easy to work with in meditation. When you say "At ease," they go "Whew."

By contrast, about half my civilian students arrive just barely on time and slightly out of breath, or even a few minutes late. They call me from their cell phones to say, "I'm stuck in traffic but I'll be right there." By inquiring how they live, I have found that they do almost everything this way. Meditation may even make them worse, because they don't really plan for the extra half hour they take in the morning to stretch and meditate. I think it is better to spend less time meditating and be early for things, so you can travel mindfully—senses open, unhurried, enjoying the ride.

At first this may sound severe, but it is really the simplest imaginable way of doing things: whatever time you say the appointment is, that is the time. Not a few minutes later or a half hour later. And because that is a simpler way of operating, it's more fun. You can even make a game out of finding out when a person is really going to arrive: you can ask, "Do you mean three, threeish, or three-thirty?" When I make appointments with people, I usually ask, "When can you realistically get there, without rushing?"

If you are early for your appointments, you can use the extra couple of minutes to collect yourself, review notes, make notes, rest, drink water, chat, take a few conscious breaths, or feel smug. More important, if you are not cutting it close, and are not late, then you will not get an adrenaline rush.

In the evening meditation, one of the things you will spend time doing is reviewing every adrenaline jolt of the day. Your body will systematically go through each nerve, soothing it and restoring it. This happens spontaneously when you relax or rest—you don't have to make it happen, and it is hard to stop it from happening, since it is a natural healing process. But it takes time in your meditation. So the fewer false alarms you have from trivial things like being late, the more time you'll have available in meditation to be with other perceptions.

If you are early for an appointment, you can cruise. You can let other people get in the elevator first; you can wave other cars ahead. You can look at people, see things, enjoy your breathing as you walk. If you feel late, the stress hormones kick in. If you have any control at all over your life, arrange to be early for everything for a month and notice how many little moments open up.

I am emphasizing this point because lots of "advanced" meditators I know have a tendency to be a little late, to chronically rush around slightly out-of-breath. It's okay to do this once in a while, or in an emergency, but it's stupid to do it habitually. Why bother to meditate, then jerk your nerves around pointlessly? Yet a huge number of meditators do this. They meditate a bit longer than they have time for, then rush out of the house and zoom to work.

The Arrive Early for Everything exercise is also good for beginning meditators. A major obstacle for most people is finding the time to meditate, and finding the time flows from having a sense of control over the rhythm of one's day. To make the space you need for meditation, you have to think backward from the time you need to walk out the door in the morning and add the extra time so you can move with leisure. You may have to get up a little earlier, which means you may have to go to bed a little earlier, which means you may have to watch less TV or enlist the cooperation of your family.

Consider experimenting with arriving early sometime.

PAUSE ON EACH THRESHOLD

TIME: 3 seconds.

Pay attention to your body, especially your belly and midline torso, when stepping across any boundary—any doorway, any entrance, any border between one space and another. You can call this a "body scan," this process of taking a quick survey of how you feel and what your senses report.

As you move through your day, you can use any threshold as a moment of awakening. Pause at any doorway, even an open door, and take a conscious breath, instead of blasting in. Notice the quality of feeling on the border (the threshold) and as you enter. Over time you will develop a physical intuition about what has been going on in the room. If you are already intuitive, this practice may help you keep your intuition sharp.

If there are people in the room, that brief pause will give them the feeling that you respect their space. The pause also lets you "catch up with yourself" as you enter.

If you are in an open space or room, you may be able to feel layers of borders around other people. All animals have zones around them. When you are a certain number of feet away from them, they are just aware of you; any closer and they get restless or alert, ready to flee (or, sometimes, attack); and then when you get too close, they move. You have invaded their space. Awareness of the invisible zones around people and animals is an intense source of joy in life.

Boundaries are flexible, because people let themselves be crowded together at times, and yet at other times they seek greater distance. At parties sometimes it is fun to be in the crowd, then you may want to go off with one person and be at a distance from the others. Lovers may at times want to merge and mingle their essence, but the whole process of relationship is one of developing appreciation for boundaries and working out the rhythms of contact and withdrawal.

Being healthy in meditation depends on respecting your own boundaries, your own limits and preferences, your yes-and-no structure. When you learn to enjoy your boundaries and be balanced within them, then the possibility of experiencing a larger boundary arises.

There are moments here and there in meditation that seem "boundless." For instance, in a breathing meditation, sometimes you may feel intimate with the ocean of air embracing the planet and embracing your body. In fact, if you pursue meditation, it is almost inevitable that you will have experiences of boundlessness. This makes it all the more important to develop your appreciation and respect for boundaries, as well as to witness the kinds of contact that occur on borders. Start by observing the feelings in your body as you cross thresholds.

TAKE A CONSCIOUS NAP

TIME: 5 minutes to 20 minutes.
PLACE: Anywhere you can be undisturbed.

Anytime you feel an energy slump or just need to change gears, you can take a conscious nap. All you do is put your head on your desk, or lie down on a bed or the floor, and pretend to nap. You may drift; you may or may not nod off. The main thing you are "doing" is recognizing and giving in to the calling of your body. You don't care whether you fall asleep or not.

Usually we resist these callings and instead think about getting another cup of tea or something to eat, or we just let our minds wander. But it is very powerful to simply give in to the sensations of fatigue and sleepiness and let them carry you wherever. You might be more relaxed if you have a clock in sight or can set an alarm so that you know you'll wake up at a certain time if you do fall asleep.

Many people have reported that after meditating for even a few days, their experience of napping changes and becomes delightful. The naps often feel even more special and sacred than the meditations. Some people prefer to "nap" rather than meditate, and they have more profound experiences in these naps than they ever do in formal meditations! Almost everyone, at certain times, needs to nap instead of doing his or her regular meditation.

One of the side effects of doing sensual meditations is that common, everyday experiences acquire an enhanced quality. Meditation trains you to notice and enjoy quiet little phenomena that are always there, and these small pleasures pop up in unexpected places.

BE COZY

TIME: About 30 minutes.

PLACE: Your nest, or anywhere special and quiet.

Choose a favorite book, magazine, tape, or CD and make a special time to be with it. Set aside at least twenty minutes; half an hour is better. Turn off the phone, put a note on the door that you are not to be disturbed, and cozy up with your favorite thing in a secluded, private spot. The idea is that you are taking good care of yourself and are natural. Part of coziness and also the next exercise, Experience Perfect Safety, is the feeling that your boundaries will be respected.

While you are reading or listening, notice your natural attention span without interfering in any way. Follow the rhythms of attention as you would when you are just being with yourself.

In the natural course of things, if you were reading or listening to something you loved, and you suddenly thought of a friend you hadn't seen in years, you might jump up and call her or him. Or you might look up from the book and just daydream. If you are listening to music, you might dance sometimes and other times lie down and close your eyes. Be that natural with yourself now, and always, when you meditate.

Notice the difference between reading in a coffee shop or airport or mall and reading at home or in another private place. Which do you prefer? Or do you have moods and sometimes prefer one situation and sometimes another?

Most people have moods and vary in what they want. One day they like reading a newspaper or book in public; another time they relish being alone. There is no need to make your meditation practice the domain of just one of your moods, to meditate only when you are happy or energetic, or when you are sad, pensive, or tired. There is no need to be so narrow in your interpretation of what meditation is. In practice, what this means is that you should eventually have three or four different types of meditations to match each of your moods—just as you may have different kinds of music or clothes to match your moods.

EXPERIENCE PERFECT SAFETY

TIME: 20 minutes.
PLACE: Somewhere quiet and protected.

If you live in the industrialized world, you are safer than 99 percent of all humanity that has ever lived, and you are statistically more likely to die from the stress you put yourself under than from any external physical threat. This statement may totally contradict what you think of as common sense—many of us are convinced by television news and other gossip that we are in mortal danger from all manner of things every time we step out of our homes. The news does a good job of screaming about the dangers that befall one person in a million, but it tells us nothing about what we will experience when we walk out the door, except maybe the weather.

Imagine a situation in which you are perfectly safe—or at least very safe. You could be anywhere in the real world or the imaginary world: in a cave underground or in the mountains; in your own special garden or on your own private island. Go ahead, build that castle in the sky, dream that dream. Then give your physical body a chance to soak up the feeling.

Review your senses. How do you breathe when you feel safe? When you look around the world, how do you absorb color when you are feeling safe? Simply explore the way your senses work when you are feeling safe in the world. Stay there and let your senses organize themselves around safety. You may feel a sense of expansion, relaxation, relief. Now visualize moving around in your current, everyday world with that sense of safety. What happens?

After a while, unsafe sensations may rise to the surface to be processed. Be with them. This is healing, so allow the process. Or if you are as snug as can be in your safe zone, let your senses drink in the feeling.

People vary so widely that it is impossible to generalize. Some people can tolerate every kind of human thought impulse with little difficulty. For them, watching thoughts is like watching TV or a movie or a stage show. Some people are at home, more or less, with every human impulse.

Other people are frightened by their thoughts and feel they have to control them. If you are this way, then do things that make you feel safe. You might want to meditate with a group in a religious context or get psychotherapy. You can do dance therapy, theater training, or journal-writing classes, and you can meditate in the physical quiet and shelter of a church. Respect your need for safety, and be gradual and gentle with yourself. If you need help with safety, get it.

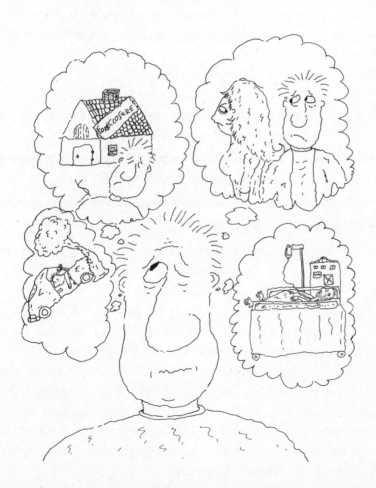

TAKE A HOT–COLD SHOWER

TIME: An extra 5 minutes in the shower (if that).

Take a hot or warm shower. Slowly turn the water on cold.

For some of us, our time in the bathroom each morning is the only quiet time of the day. If that's true for you, make the shower a sanctuary. Bathing in the morning before work is usually a habitual set of motions. You had to make it that way at some point in your past in order to get to work on time. Now you have that handled and you're an adult; you have the right to enjoy your body while you are bathing.

All you have to do in the beginning is move more slowly. You do that because it is easier to be attentive when you are moving with less haste. After you get used to paying attention, you can move quickly and still be attentive.

Some ideas of sensual things to attend to:

- Have good things to smell, perhaps several types of body shampoo. Breathe in the smell while shampooing.
- Take longer with your head under the water. Enjoy some conscious breaths with the water streaming over your hair.
- Let the water massage your neck while you breathe consciously.
- Take longer shaving or toweling.
- Rub lotion all over your body. (It is a very different experience to rub lotion on skin that has been chilled slightly.)

After you have gotten into that, perhaps after a few days, experiment with turning the water on cool at the end. Do that for a few days, then gradually make the water cooler and cooler.

Cold is refreshing. It makes the skin tingle and, if gotten used to gradually, is very healthy. The human body can easily handle cold; just be gradual, and proceed only in accord with your pleasure. It can take a month to be able to handle a cold shower even for ten seconds and have it be pleasurable. Yet it is an amazing wake-up that makes you very aware of your skin as a boundary.

Embracing the cold also trains the body to thrive on being shocked. You are there in the shower, luxuriating, and then the cold comes on. As you get used to it gradually, the shock becomes invigorating rather than painful. And we all need help in gracefully meeting the shocks that life provides.

Then, awakened, stand there and bless everyone you will meet that day. Send light and love ahead of you along the path you will walk.

When you walk out of the bathroom, toweling yourself off, you will be ready for the day.

If you have time for a longer meditation, this self-care will help prepare the body for relaxed alertness. Some people, for example, work out or do yoga for forty-five minutes, then shower, then meditate.

DO THE SLUMP

TIME: A minute or two.

WHERE: At your desk or anywhere else.

Let your spine curl forward and your head drop slowly. Feel the weight of your shoulders as they slump forward, and notice the curve of your back. There is a gentle stretch all the way from your waist, through your entire spine, to your neck.

Stay there for a moment and breathe, and extend the stretch as long as you like.

All you are doing is letting your upper body give in to gravity. Luxuriate in the feeling of not having to hold yourself up. Gravity is the masseur.

Then, very slowly, come back to an erect posture. Savor the sensations all over your body. You may have sensations in your skull, a feeling of relief, a tingling through your back, and other pleasurable kinesthetics (bodily sensations of movement).

You can do this exercise over and over again, as much as you like.

It is also a great exercise to do at the beginning and end of every meditation.

GIVE IN TO GRAVITY

TIME: 5 minutes.
WHERE: Anywhere you can get down.

You can do this exercise while sitting, standing, or lying down. Explore it in all postures and go with what feels most interesting to you.

Notice the ground beneath you. Look around you and see the foundation beneath you. Then feel the areas of your body that are in contact with that foundation.

An invisible force, centered in the Earth's core, is attracting your body to the very center of the Earth's body. This is called gravity. Although we rarely notice gravity, we have sensors in our body that constantly monitor our relationship with it.

Surrender to the downward pull of gravity while staying in your same posture. Let your senses of touch and balance become alert to the pull of gravity. Gravity is not just heaviness; gravity is *attraction*. And attraction is always interesting. Gravity is a form of love.

If you are standing, stay erect but let your body hang off your bones. I know this sounds strange, but that's the way the skeleton is designed: all those bones hold you up. Your muscles can let go.

If you are sitting, either in a chair with your feet on the ground or with your butt on the ground and your feet tucked up, then sit upright as you let your pelvis be pulled by gravity into a snug contact with the Earth.

If you are lying down, then completely let go, let yourself drop, and feel the way the Earth holds you up.

In all postures, no matter how much you let yourself go and surrender to gravity, the Earth supports you. You do not fall through the floor.

But it sometimes feels as if your consciousness falls through the floor and touches some energy core inside the Earth. This is a very simple experience even though it takes many words to describe it. It is as though some part of yourself reaches down, like a root, and taps into a source of energy and power originating in Nature. Indian, Tibetan, and Chinese yoga masters talk of an energy center between the legs, which they call the "root center." This center comes alive when you surrender to gravity; it sparkles and tingles, and you may feel energy coming into your body and moving down your legs.

Once you give in to gravity, simply enjoy the sensations and breathe.

Stay there for a while, and you will begin to feel lighter and lighter. Having surrendered to gravity, you make friends with it. Your body reorganizes itself and begins to experience gravity as a force holding you up as much as a force pulling you down.

NOTICE WHAT'S UP?

TIME: 1 minute to 5 minutes.
WHERE: Indoors or outside.
WHEN: Sometime when the sun is up.

Standing or sitting, raise your arms above your head and notice what is there. Notice how "up" feels. What does the space above your head feel like?

Solar power comes from above, and when people think of their Higher Power, they often think of it as above. Perhaps because of this natural feeling of a source overhead, we can actually reach into the Above and bring its blessing down into our bodies.

Hold your hands out, as if embracing the sky, reaching upward to the sky in celebration or greeting.

You could also explore turning your palms to face each other as you hold your arms over your head. Pay attention to any sensations of currents flowing between the hands.

Then, slowly, let the hands drift downward and almost touch the top of the head; pause and breathe, then lightly touch the head.

Move the hands upward again, pause for a moment with the arms extended, then bring the hands slowly down and almost touch the heart area; pause, then lightly touch.

Tip: The first time you do this exercise, give yourself fifteen minutes when you are relaxed and, preferably, outdoors. Do the movements extremely slowly and with playful ease. Do the movements over and over so that your body becomes accustomed to them, and so that you can get used to detecting the subtle pleasurable sensations.

After you become familiar with these movements, you may find that you can experience the effect in a few seconds.

Reach up again, pause, then bring the hands down to almost touch the belly; pause there, then lightly touch.

Savor the flow of power downward from the Higher Power or the sun, through your body, into the Earth.

If you want, you could take a moment to linger with any pleasurable sensations on the top of your head, in your heart, or in your belly.

TENSE TO RELAX

TIME: 1 minute to 5 minutes.

WHERE: You can do the exercise invisibly wherever you are, or you can get down on the floor and go to town.

With the body, almost everything is done in opposites. If you want to breathe in, breathe out first. If you want to be rested and energetic tomorrow, go to sleep tonight. The situation is similar with relaxation: if you want to relax your muscles, tense them first.

Get into tensing and relaxing gradually, at your own pace. Experiment with tensing and relaxing your face, your hands and arms, your legs—you pick the body part and the sequence of movement from part to part. Voluntarily tensing your muscles is definitely *doing* something. It is an action. To relax, don't do anything and do not tell yourself to relax. Just let go of the tensing action.

Explore also the different feelings invoked when you tense for longer or shorter periods of time. Tense and hold for a certain number of breaths, then release and notice the sensations.

Experiment with tensing and relaxing while sitting up, lying down, and stretched out on the floor in various postures.

Tense your entire body, all the muscles simultaneously, then release.

Do Tense to Relax every day for several minutes, and give yourself a month to get really familiar with it.

NOTE: Tensing and relaxing is a more realistic approach to relaxation than attempting to relax directly. I am not sure what happens when people tell themselves to "relax." Do they just go limp? Relaxation is not limpness; it is the state of not having any *unnecessary* tension. As long as we are alive, the muscles are in a slight state of tension—and this is good; it is the way the muscles work. When we are excited, it is a pleasant state of readiness in the body, akin to tension, but more finely tuned. Relaxation happens naturally in meditation, as a side effect of being more perceptive and at home in ourselves. It's not something to go for directly.

LET YOUR BRAIN GO LIMP

TIME: 1 minute.

Sitting comfortably, put your palm on the back of your head, at the base of the skull. Let your head rest back into your hand and stay that way for a few breaths.

As the breath flows in and out, the wave motion creates an undulation up the spine into the skull. Enjoy this sensation for a few more breaths.

Then take away your hand and let it go limp in your lap. Now imagine your brain going limp, as though it doesn't have to work at all for the next minute.

If you have a sinking sensation, go with it—let your attention drop into your body. This is just like the Slump exercise, except that there is no outward physical movement.

Savor the feeling of relief.

FIND STILLNESS IN MOTION

TIME: 5 minutes.
WHEN: Anytime you are rested and unhurried.

Find a chair that gives you a sense of being firmly planted. Your pelvis is supported but you are free to move your torso, and your feet are on the ground. An office chair is good for this.

Let yourself rock a little in any manner, back and forth or side to side. This is the same movement people make when they are restless or can't make up their minds. The movement comes from that same instinctive place.

Let this movement segue into a circle. Your tailbone is on the seat, but upward from there your torso is orbiting around.

Stay with the circle and allow your senses of balance and motion to engage with the movement you are in. This may take anywhere from a few seconds to a minute. When it feels natural, close your eyes and continue.

NOTE: Still motion is a very worthwhile sense to cultivate. When you get it, your whole meditation practice will be enriched, and "stillness" will seem a very lively event. Give it a chance sometime—if you fall in love with it immediately, then include a little of it in your daily meditation. If it seems strange to you, return again in a week or a month and check it out again. You won't be able to do this meditation if you have had a cold or flu recently or if you are taking medication that affects the inner ear.

As you are moving, you will find your kinesthetic senses tracking the movement. Have a sense of curiosity about what you will experience, and continue.

Over a period of time, you will probably find yourself wanting to slow the movement. What you can do is let the movement coast to a stop.

Continue to track the movement and notice what happens. If your nervous system is organized enough in the moment to process the experience, the sense of motion may actually become more intense as the physical motion lessens.

As the movement coasts toward stillness, it may transform into a curiously blended sense of stillness and motion—"still motion." You will know it when you discover it, because the sensation is liquid and exquisite.

 Variation

Invisible Motion of the Head

With the eyes open, make the tiniest motion of the head you can notice. The movement could be left to right and back or a slight tilting of the chin up and down. Allow the eyes to close—or not—of their own accord as you let your senses inform you of this minute movement. (This exercise is an elaboration on the Salute to Balance.)

Continue to track the sense of motion, and notice the feelings you have in your skull and elsewhere as your attention engages with the vestibular sense and the joint sensors in the vertebrae of your neck.

You may find yourself taking a few deep breaths as your body settles into tracking mode. Delicate motion of the head is used in hunting and tracking, and the body knows well how to do it. You use the same senses to avoid becoming prey by knowing if you are being tracked. You may find yourself feeling stealthy. Your sense of hearing may open up to detect variations in the silence.

For now, return to the tiny, just-barely-noticeable differences in motion of the neck. Allow your attention to shift back and forth between those sensations and the sensation of breathing, if that is what happens naturally. Eventually, your body will quiet itself enough to notice the motion very clearly.

Explore whatever movements you want to make, in any direction.

NOTE: Meditations that involve the neck and head tend to evoke a lot of stretching. This is because paying attention to the head, without telling it what to do, gives the neck muscles permission to seek balance. Almost all movements of modern people involve leaning forward: driving, reading, sitting at a desk, child care, manual labor. You will be able to do this exercise much better after stretching.

This brings up a major point: it is good, and a success of meditation, if doing an exercise makes you feel restless. Almost all meditators think they have failed when they do a meditation for two minutes, then get restless and start stretching. But this is a major blessing. What has happened is that your body has gone into self-regeneration mode. It is wanting to invent its own yoga postures, which is what stretching is. Think about this sometime, because often what meditators consider their failure is actually a success.

Invisible motion is part of every breath—there are very slight motions of the head with every in- and outbreath, in addition to the not-so-invisible motion of the ribs expanding and contracting with the breath. Learning to appreciate these minute motions will enrich your meditative experience. Explore Stillness in Motion on its own, and give your body a chance to get used to it. Then include it in your longer meditations.

EXPLORE YOUR MAGNETIC HANDS

TIME: From 30 seconds to 5 minutes.
WHERE: Anywhere.

Sometime when you are at ease, either standing or sitting, let your hands "become aware of each other." In other words, be alert in your hands. Notice what happens over the span of a few breaths as you pay attention to your hands.

Now let the hands drift up so they are facing each other. The palms can be about a foot and a half apart and in front of the belly. Explore until you find a position that feels better than others.

Let your attention drop a bit and rest in your breath, then pay attention to the sensations in your hands or between your hands with a mild curiosity.

After you get used to being in this posture for a minute, notice what qualities of sensation you feel. What does the empty space between your hands feel like? What subtle tinglings do the palms detect?

Move your hands in an exploratory fashion, compressing the air, fluffing it. Move very slowly and notice what you sense.

Warmth?
Pressure?
A cottony sensation, as if there is something there?
Magnetism?
Tingling?

Give the exploration a couple of minutes anytime you are curious. Do not concentrate or try at all; simply be curious. If you do feel a sense of magnetism between your hands, play with it a little, then return to it tomorrow or another time.

If you don't feel anything, experiment sometime at the end of a meditation or when you feel energized.

 Variation

Sign Language

Another way in to hand sensitivity is to observe people talking with their hands. As you move through your day, notice people's spontaneous hand movements and make a mental catalog of them. If you can, talk with some Italians and hang out with deaf people talking in sign language. Then, when you are getting ready to meditate and are alone, say with your hands what you want out of meditation. Make up a prayer in your own talking-with-the-hands language. Say how you feel now and then say how you want to feel after meditation. You may not be able to say verbally what you want, but you may be able to dance it with hand and arm motions.

Variation

Rowing the Air

Sitting or standing, draw your hands in toward your chest as you breathe in, and move them away from the chest as you breathe out. Experiment with different distances, just doing what feels slightly pleasurable.

The palms can be turned in toward you through both movements, or you can turn them to face outward when you breathe out.

Let the arms and hands be at ease as you move, the elbows down, the forearms pointing up slightly.

Someday when you want to, play with this exercise for about five minutes. Often that is how long it takes to get used to the movement so that your sensory system can feel the energetic charge building up.

You may feel "something" there between your hands and your chest, something coming into your chest and flowing around. It may feel like the essence of vitality, as when you are at the ocean or among green trees and breathe.

Your hands may become tingly and magnetic, and your heart may feel washed with sparkling air-stuff. An amazing number of people are sensitive to this subtle energy. Sometimes I'll have fifty people in a room do this exercise, and forty of them immediately begin sensing the energy. Since you are on your own, the trick is to be informal with yourself. Sneak up on yourself at different times and check in with what you feel with motion and breath. If and when you awaken to this sensitivity, it will make your breath-awareness meditations that much more interesting.

With new groups and veteran meditators alike, I often walk into the room and have them do this exercise without the slightest preparation or warning. They don't even have time to think about whether they will do it right. I like to listen to what people say as they start perceiving the energy flowing, whether it is between their palms in the Magnetic Hands exercise or between the palms and the heart in the Rowing Air exercise. Everyone is standing around saying things like, Hmmm . . . warm . . . magnetic . . . empty space feels like substance . . . sort of plasma, charged particles . . . feels like a ball of light.

Remember—discover, don't impose. If you don't feel anything today, just explore this technique next week, and at a different time of day, or after you have done a different meditation. Or forget about it altogether! Do not judge yourself. There is no one language, no one technique that speaks to everyone.

BEFORE-SLEEP MEDITATIONS

TIME: 5 minutes.

WHERE: Sitting or lying in bed.

Using your senses of motion and touch, enjoy the flow of breathing for a few minutes as you are getting ready for sleep. You can sit up in bed, then slide down under the covers; or you can do the whole thing lying down. Go with whatever your preference is.

Invite the feeling of drifting, since you are intending to drift off into sleep. If your nerves are jangled, you can meditate on the quality of "soothing" or "peace."

Sometimes the simplest things are the most neglected. Before-bed meditations cost no money and probably won't take any time out of your evening except away from the television or a book. The basic idea is to treat yourself as you would at a health spa. You'd turn in early, maybe as early as 9:00 P.M., and have no television. Maybe just a peaceful book to read and a candle.

The next morning, notice how you feel. Are you more rested? More relaxed and ready for the day? Give this three days as an experiment sometime soon. Then, if you like it, continue.

An hour or so before bed, you might want to bathe or shower and, even if you are a man, massage your whole body with a light moisturizer or lotion. This will help the body shift gears into rest mode.

If you usually drink alcohol at night, drink herbal tea or water instead. If you never drink at night, try half a glass of wine sometime.

Do a little stretching—very light, just enough to evoke a languorous feeling. Then go to bed early and welcome the process of letting your mind drift. You might review the day, or you might find yourself planning a vacation or remodeling the kitchen. It doesn't matter. What does matter is that you set your mind free.

When people go camping, one of the healing elements is absence of electric light and an early bedtime. Under those conditions it's not unusual to wake up during the night and gaze at the stars for a while before drifting off again. During the night, campers often spend a lot of time sleepily meditating under the canopy of stars. This is a very renewing and balancing process. When you are at home, you can turn off the bright lights, have just a dim light, and begin to shift into rest mode more gradually than you usually do. You might find you love the gradualness.

You can also spruce up your sleeping space. Look around it in the evening and notice what you want to do to make it a more inviting place. Do what you can, and over time keep paying attention to the space in and around your bed.

Bed can be a sanctuary. Lots of spiritual people neglect the bed as sanctuary, as if it is more sacred somehow to sit on a wooden floor in the next room. Well, more power to them. But we all spend about a third of our lives in bed, or else suffer from lack of rest. So it is a very worthwhile sanctuary to cultivate.

Over time, you will pay off your sleep debt, both through getting more sleep and through having a deeper sleep. Then you will be more able to enjoy the transitions—from waking to sleeping and from sleeping to waking. Transitions are exquisite, magical times. You can learn a lot about meditation by witnessing transitions between states of consciousness.

Moreover, as you pay off your sleep debt, you will begin awakening naturally in the morning, without an alarm and feeling fresher. You may even find that you have time to meditate as soon as you start to flicker into wakefulness, and this is a delightful thing to do, to just lie there savoring existence before even opening your eyes.

Take as long as you like to develop your preferences and habits in approaching sleep. All you need to remember is to treat yourself well and have a gradual phasing in to sleep. I have been doing various before-sleep meditations for more than twenty years, and I am still discovering new things.

Last year, I started visualizing the Earth from space while falling asleep. I wanted to have a sense of falling into the universe as I fell asleep. It took a few weeks for the visualization to be completely automatic and effortless, and then I found I had my favorite viewpoint—right over the Pacific, looking into that deep blue.

There are many fantastic photographs of the Earth from space and space from the Hubble telescope. I recommend finding some you are particularly taken with and looking at them before you fall asleep.

Make Yourself Comfortable

Give before-sleep meditations two weeks, and notice how they affect your sleep and your waking hours. Sleep is a time to let your soul fly free. Consider exposing your attention to the vastness and beauty of the universe as you get ready for sleep.

Make friends with the dark. Often there is some sort of light in the bedroom—a VCR with its glowing clock, light streaming through a window. Consider making the bedroom completely dark by devising some sort of blackout covers for the windows. Then welcome the experience of darkness; it is very restful and will tend to make you appreciate the light that much more when it comes time to awaken.

REVIEW OF THE DAY

TIME: 10 minutes.
WHEN: Toward the end of the day.

Few of us are able to move through a day and finish every conversation, give full attention and expression to every emotion, check off every item on our list, and adequately appreciate all the people around us. There is always something unfinished, more to feel, more to realize.

By consciously and intentionally giving yourself a time to review the day before going to sleep, you help to unburden your sleep time from having to deal with this unfinished business.

How to do it: Spend a minute or two settling in, then review your day either from the beginning to the end or by working backward from where you are now to the time you awoke this morning. Touch upon all areas of concern, anything that worried you or felt incomplete. Also remember the moments of pleasure, and give yourself time to feel gratitude for what you have.

If you have had a challenging day, you may want to extend your settling-in time, to relax more before beginning the review.

This simple, almost invisible practice of reviewing the day can dramatically improve the quality of your life. Many people do it naturally, and don't even think of it as meditation, yet it blesses their lives. Many other people I meet used to do something like this until a new job, a new relationship, a new baby, or some other life event made their quiet time disappear. Years later, they notice a feeling of missing something and finally realize that they are no longer giving themselves time to sit with themselves and be grateful, not even ten minutes a day.

It is easy to get swept up in being so busy that we forget to take time for quiet moments to reflect on what the day has brought.

HEART-CENTERED MEDITATIONS

TIME: 1 minute to 10 minutes.

WHEN: Anytime you have heartache or joy that needs attending to.

Sometime when you are relatively quiet inside, let attention rest in the area around the physical heart and lungs. The lungs are spacious and the heart is muscular. Corresponding to those physical organs is an area of *pure feeling*. This feeling center is what people informally refer to when they say that their heart aches or their heart is glad.

To get into that feeling center, recall some great experience that made your heart glad, that made you glad to be alive. Just thinking of it will cause a sensation to arise in your heart—it could be a sense of light or swelling, an upward-moving current of electricity, or a vibration. Use that sensation as a homing signal and let attention be called into that place called "the heart." Be alert, because the sensations may last for only a flash, a few seconds.

As attention rests there, become aware also of the gentle pulsing of breath.

If you are experiencing sorrow or grief, you may already have sensations in the heart. If so, simply be with them. The sensations are calling you.

You may also have a sense of joy and gratitude about events in your life, and may have wonderful sensations in your heart center. We can neglect to pay attention to our joy, just as we can neglect adequately to be with our pain.

If you do not have sensations or feelings of ache or joy in the heart, don't worry. Someday you will. Come back then to this exercise and check it out.

If at some point while meditating, you find strong emotions going through you, explore this simple practice of resting attention in the heart.

As you breathe in and out, be alert to the qualities of emotion you are feeling. If you are feeling an emotion, be aware that it may change every couple of minutes into something else. Sometimes the emotions change every few seconds. They may include:

Comfort
Relief
Sorrow
Peacefulness
Happiness
Anger
Hurt
Excitement

Go back from the sternum, inward. Feel all the way back to the spine. That is the heart area.

Simply being with these sensations will help tremendously, for the heart knows how to heal itself and become available to love again. You have only to willingly tolerate the aching.

When you "speak from the heart" you are speaking from inside those sensations. Courage is "to have heart." To stay in the heart when you are afraid or the sensations are too much to bear, but you bear them anyway—that is the definition of courage. As you breathe in, the world is touching you, renewing you, encouraging (en-courage-ing) you to live again, adventure forth, and experience.

 Variations

Greet and Say Good-bye

Here is a simple approach to a heart meditation:

Be there in the heart to greet the incoming breath. Embrace it. Be awake to the gift that life is giving you with this breath.

Say good-bye to the outgoing breath. Let go of it. Be awake to the freedom that comes from letting go of the old air, old thoughts, old feelings.

Expansion and Contraction

Notice that as you breathe in, you expand to encompass the incoming breath.

On the physical level, your rib cage and torso expand.

Tolerate the experience of that expansion continuing.
Savor the sense of expansion evoked by the flow of breath.

As you breathe in, your rib cage expands outward from your center to embrace the new air. With your attention, embrace the new life.

As you breathe in, your being expands to encompass the world.

Be there in the heart as the breath flows in.
Be awake to the gift life is giving you.

Getting into Breath

Breath has sound and texture and motion. As your body moves with the inflowing and outflowing breath, your body balances automatically. Breath even has an impact on the visual field, producing subtle differences that you can notice.

Breathing with awareness is one of the essential meditation techniques cherished the world over. Simply pay attention to the flow of air with appreciation for the gift of each breath. Doing this even a few minutes a day will bless your life. Human beings develop senses for whatever they pay attention to. If you pay a lot of attention to wine, you will learn to identify what type it is just by a sniff of the bouquet. If you watch a lot of baseball, you will learn to see what type of pitch is coming earlier and earlier in the wind-up or release. Mothers can tell the state of their babies at a glance. If you pay attention to breath, your body will over time evolve the senses to really, really enjoy it as one of the Fine Things of Life.

Breath has to be mostly automatic and out-of-awareness by default, because our life depends on it every minute. We breathe many times a minute, whether we are awake or asleep. In a day we breathe more than twenty thousand times. Each of these breaths connects us to the entire planet. Appreciating this connection is joyous but optional—it is what we do after survival is assured.

The movement of attention to cherish breath is instinctive, for all living things have a natural attraction toward that which gives them life. Meditation is an instinctive urge, a calling as deep as any of the ancient yearnings that move human beings. All the hundreds of techniques are just ways of cooperating with that urge. For meditation to feel innate, it helps to learn it at your own speed in your own way. Start now. Take a breath, have fun.

TAKE A BREATHER

If you feel like it, take a minute right now to explore what you enjoy about breath. Instead of "concentrating" on the breath, take a wondering and exploring attitude toward your relationship with breath. Breath will teach you how to pay attention to it.

For example, think of some of the times in your life when you have found yourself appreciating the action of breathing.

- Walking outside on a snowy morning and seeing the air you exhale turn into a mist.
- When in nature, coming to a vista and taking a deep breath to breathe in the beauty.
- Saying "Whew" at a moment of relief.
- Yawning and stretching with a deep inhalation.
- Saying "Ah . . ." as you exhale and settle down into yourself.
- Playing sports.
- Panting during sex.
- Inhaling a delicious smell and saying "Mmmmmm . . ."
- Finishing a task, leaning back, and sighing with relief.

Take a few moments to recall three or four times you have said "Ah" or "Whew" or "Mmmmmm." Then for a minute or two, simply notice the pleasure of breathing. You can have your eyes open or closed or go back and forth.

If you are having a good time, you can continue for another minute or two. Simply notice what happens in your body as you pay attention to the flow of air in and out.

As you pay attention to breathing, a whole world of sensory experience will gradually unfold.

- The beginning impulse to inhale.
- The air flowing in through the nose.
- The air flowing up the nose into the sinuses.
- The silky sensation of air flowing down the throat.
- The air filling the lungs, deep in the body.
- The brief pause at the end of the inhalation as the breath turns to flow out.
- The relief of breath flowing out.
- The pause at the end of the exhalation as breath turns to flow in.

Other qualities of experience that emerge are:

- The rhythm of the breath.
- The smell of the air. Maybe there is a flower nearby, or someone is cooking.
- The motion and undulation of the body as the ribs expand into the inbreath and contract with the outbreath.
- The quiet sound of the air flowing and whispering through the same passages we use to sing and talk.

If your eyes are open, you may also notice the way the eyes tend to rest on one spot when you are focused on breathing. You can then let the peripheral vision open up to take in a larger view.

> ◎ **Tip:** There is no hurry. Take your time. I have met many people who have taken an earnest, diligent approach to learning yoga breathing techniques. The problem is that the attitude can persist. Years later, breath is still something to be controlled. Enjoy your breath. If you explore, you will find what you enjoy, in your own sweet time.

The more senses you allow to come into play during meditation, the more interesting and involving your experience will become.

A wine taster can take a sniff of wine, then a sip, and say what kind of wine it is and perhaps where it was grown and when. You can learn to have that appreciative attitude and richness of experience with your own breath.

With each breath, you import substance from the ocean of air that embraces the Earth, and you give back to the world the substance you have already used.

WELCOME A BREATH

In this meditation you take the attitude of actively welcoming breath. You do not need to control it in any way.

Standing or sitting, turn to face any direction you like and welcome the inflowing breath. Lean forward slightly, leaning into the breath. Greet the air as you would a beloved guest coming into your home. Allow your thoughts to come and go, but keep bringing your attention back to the encounter with breath.

You can have any attitude you want, or you may find yourself moving from attitude to attitude as you pay attention:

> Restlessness
> Curiosity
> Wonder
> Gratitude
> Relief
> Sensual pleasure

If you like, say to yourself, "This breath is the breath of my being."

The breath is a gift to you from the entire history of the world: all the oceans, all the forests, the sun. Each time you breathe in, the whole world and all of history is coming into your body to keep you alive for a few more moments. Each time you breathe, the mystery of the sun shining on the oceans and forests of the world comes into your lungs. The lungs are temples for receiving the spirit of the universe. A secret of meditation is that the universe is sensuously intimate in its vastness. This is a secret that every breath is eager to share with you.

Be as natural with yourself as you are when you spontaneously sigh or yawn. Notice your relationship with breathing, and take pleasure in it.

Place your attention on each of the following for a few seconds:

Rest the attention on the flow of breath in your body.

As you breathe in, notice the sensations of expansion.

Attend to breath as a flow from the whole world into your body. Be aware that the ocean of air giving you life is something that it took a whole planet and the sun eons to produce. Be aware of all the oceans of the world as you breathe.

Be aware of the sun shining continuously on the Earth as you follow the flow of breathing in your body.

Now place your attention in the middle of the chest—not on the surface, but deep inside, in the space you breathe into. Welcome the breath from there. Celebrate the way the incoming air flows into those deep spaces inside you, refreshing you.

YAWN TO WAKE UP

TIME: Anywhere from 15 seconds to 5 minutes.

WHEN: Anytime you find yourself wanting to yawn, get into it as much as you can. Prolong the stretches and deep inhalations.

When we neglect yawning, we miss out on a great human activity. It is spontaneous—the body just does it. It takes less than a minute, and it's refreshing.

If it is natural for you to do so right now, let yourself yawn or stretch or sigh. If not now, then the next time you have a chance, give over to a yawn completely and without hurry. Adults almost never really indulge yawning, and yet it is a personal and spontaneous form of yoga. It is where yoga came from.

When you have some time—perhaps in the morning or in the evening after work when you want to meditate—really get into yawning. Spend five minutes stretching every way you want.

Yawn for a while and learn about how your body likes to breathe. You will learn a lot.

A yawn is a stretch in the jaw. It may lead to a full-body stretch. Get down on the floor and let yourself stretch. See if you can invent stretches for two minutes. Your body will teach you a great deal about yoga in those two minutes.

You can do Yawn to Wake Up in combination with the tense-and-relax exercise. Yawning is the source of Tense to Relax—and of yoga in general.

BREATHE FAST

TIME: 10 seconds to 5 minutes.

WHEN: At beginning or end of meditation.

Fast breath during meditation has some of the exciting qualities of fast cars and fast horses. It can wake you up and clear your head.

Here is a simple breath exercise. Have a watch at hand or a clock within sight.

For ten seconds, breathe rapidly in and out through your nose, with the mouth closed.

Notice how you feel. Scan your head and your senses.

Then continue breathing rapidly for another twenty seconds.

Notice how you feel.

If you enjoy the sensation, do another minute of fast breathing.

Obviously, do not do this if you are driving. But it is very safe to breathe rapidly. People breathe like this when they are exercising, dancing, making love, climbing stairs, running. It is very energizing. Don't worry about hyperventilating. The body is extremely good at balancing oxygen levels in the blood. If you have any concerns, though, do not do it.

If you are on medication for high blood pressure or have a chronic illness, don't do this meditation. But if you can exercise, then you can breathe fast.

Over a period of weeks, explore fast breathing before and after your meditation sessions, or as a thing in itself. Give your body a chance to become at home with it.

EXHALE SLOWLY

TIME: 1 minute.

WHERE: Anywhere.

Take a deep breath, feeling the expansion of your chest outward in all directions. Then exhale normally.

Take another deep breath, but this time exhale very slowly, letting just the smallest stream of breath flow out. Feel the place in your throat that you can constrict if you want to whisper. Use that place to gently restrict the flow of breath. Get used to that constriction, and notice that your breath makes a slight sound, a soft *hhhhh* or *ahhh*.

You can exhale either through the mouth or through the nose. Do whichever you prefer.

As you exhale, feel the slow deflation of your chest. That's all. Continue for as long as you like.

Get used to this very simple breath and explore it under many conditions. When you become comfortable with it, you may find that you can use it to change gears in the space of a few breaths. You can use it almost anywhere, under almost any conditions.

It is very relaxing and comforting, and it helps to dissolve tension. It creates a feeling of melting and spreading.

INHALE AND HOLD A BREATH

TIME: 5 minutes.

WHERE: It's good to do outside.

Inhale slightly more than usual and hold the breath for a few seconds. Then exhale normally. Do this again and again, and pay attention to the top of your head.

Then settle into a normal breathing pattern, neither deep nor shallow. At the end of each inhalation, hold for a brief moment. Continue to be alert to sensations in the top of the head.

Over time, as you get used to this pause, you will develop the senses to notice when you are coming to the end of an inhalation. Then you can glide to the end. It is like taking your foot off the accelerator and coasting before braking and entering a turn. It's a natural movement you can fall into.

◎ Variation

Just for a moment at the end of the inhalation, attention lights upon a blessed place in the crown of the skull. There is no effort or focusing, only the simple act of touching that place with attention.

Think of the greatest thing in the world—the moment of orgasm, or perfect peace, or the most beautiful sunlight, or someone you love, or the highest desire you have.

Pay attention to the overall feel of your body. Notice what happens as you pause for a moment on the inhalation.

This breath is probably the instinctive origin of tobacco and marijuana smoking. Something as popular as those activities has to have a foundation in a natural movement of the body. We crave the experience of something special in the incoming breath. So why not just let ourselves satisfy this craving with plain old air?

Yogis have always recommended savoring breath and occasionally pausing at the end of inhalation or exhalation.

BREATHE POWER

TIME: 10 seconds.

WHEN: Anytime.

As you move through your day, you can call on any quality you want by thinking its name as you take in a conscious breath. The trick is to allow yourself to feel your desire or your need for the quality. Then attention will naturally be on that quality as you breathe. Necessity is the mother of invention.

The first few times you do this, you may want to be relaxed and have a lot of time.

Experiment now. Be awake in your body for some quality of feeling you crave or desire. Then simply be aware of that quality as you breathe in.

Power

Relief

Love

Peace

Centeredness

Alertness

Calm

Inspiration

Energy

Notice that the qualities can be opposites—energy and calmness, for example. Breath is opposites. You breathe in fresh air and energy and you breathe out old air and tension.

If you want to get rid of feelings or thoughts (purification), pay attention to the breath flowing out.

If you want energy and inspiration, pay attention to the breath flowing in.

More effective than thinking the *name* of the quality is *feeling* it. Some people can refer to a feeling immediately without words. Other people find it easier with words, and still others use images or colors.

Check out this exercise and see if it works for you. If it doesn't work right away, experiment with it next week, and the week after.

One way in for this exercise is to get into it sometime when you are in a magical moment—watching a sunset or sunrise, communing with nature, enjoying a good walk. Once you are at home with the exercise, you can call on it as needed.

This exercise is as good when done for a few seconds here and there during the day as it is when part of a longer meditation.

BREATHE THE BREATH OF LIFE

Love, communion, nourishment, vastness, terror, and ecstasy are there in every breath. To experience this right now, just breathe out and don't breathe in for a few seconds. . . . Go ahead, breathe out and then pause before breathing in and notice what happens.

Stay with the pause as long as you want.

When you finally breathe in, pay attention to the sensation or world of sensations. What is it? Let the sense of relief unfold into its various subqualities. Play around with pausing briefly at the end of both inhalation and exhalation. Which is your favorite, the pause at the end of exhalation or the pause at the end of inhalation? Or is it the middle part of the breath, the smoothly flowing caress of air? Take another moment to explore your sensuous experience of breath, no matter how tiny the sensations are.

You have just experienced how totally dependent you are on Earth's ecosystem for each molecule of air that you breathe. You will die within minutes if you just stop breathing, and right there is terror enough, implicit if not explicit. Every breath that you or anyone else has ever breathed is an unconscious prayer to the totality of the world, a statement of your fundamental connectedness with every cell of algae in every ocean, every plant on all the continents, every wave-like particle of sunlight that touches the Earth. Air circulates so freely that each breath contains molecules that have passed through the lungs and heart of every creature that has ever lived—Buddha, Jesus, and the tyrannosaur whose bones stand in the museum.

Meditation is this simple and immediate. In fact, the most important and basic of all meditation techniques is to notice what it is to breathe. There are many hundreds of meditative breath techniques, but the essence is to inquire, What is it to breathe? Then let your senses awaken and take you on an inner journey of discovery. Although many expert meditators have inquired in this way over the past four thousand or so years, many more just regular folks have gone the same route. I think it began many tens of thousands of years ago, whenever human beings had a few quiet moments in the cave or savanna and enough language to talk about it.

Meditation is not an intellectual pursuit but rather the pursuit of rich experience and the full development of the experiencer. It is sensuous and vivid and relational. So the answer to the question of what is breath is not an answer that can come in words. The answer is what happens to you when you learn to cherish breath day in and day out over a period of months and years.

The answer lies in the way the world opens up in wonderful ways. All the senses are enhanced, and a spontaneous reverence emerges for the world and the space around it. I constantly meet people who secretly practice this kind of attentiveness. They do not even think of it as meditation; it is just a mystery they are exploring, a secret love affair they are having with the life force. They are invariably surprised to learn that they already know how to do a basic form of meditation. True, there is always more to learn, but the essential approach that we call meditation is something most human beings are already adept at in some small way, in their best moments. The task is to take those best moments and extend them.

There is little about meditation that one could not learn by being attentive to what it is to be in love—not just romantic love but everyday love, the kind of love that spans years and decades. A person who loves deeply and has learned to be true to the demands of relationship may know as much about meditation as someone who has spent years in a cave. Meditation is a surrender to love's forces, letting ourselves be molded by that which is the greatest in us. The recluse in the cave is surrendering to her wild and passionate love for the vastness of space and silence. That is not a more spiritual passion than some other kind of love; it is just a different context for surrendering.

You may as well choose from among the meditations presented here the ones you can fall in love with. This is different for everyone, and even for the same person it changes over time, like musical taste. Every now and then, meditators have to go on hunting expeditions for their next passion in meditation. There is no point in doing breath meditations unless you are willing to be entertained by breath and even risk falling in love with the process.

Getting into Sound

Sound, like breath, is infinitely interesting. Think of how much music of all types, live and recorded, is being played and broadcast around the world at this moment. On every continent music is being played because human beings like to listen to melodic sounds. People are making sounds with every kind of instrument: stringed instruments, breath instruments such as the flute, percussion instruments, electronic instruments that can imitate anything, and the human voice.

To use sound in meditation, start from where you are with sound, then learn to listen to progressively quieter sounds until you are listening to silence. At that moment you may experience a moment of mental silence as well. Although brief, those moments are immensely refreshing. The world does not have to become still for you to experience silence. There is a stillness underneath sound that is there for anyone to partake in.

If you are in nature right now, there may be sounds you can use as a focus: a waterfall, a brook, the wind in the trees. If you are in your home or at work, there are probably numerous sounds in the background. The hum of refrigerators, computers, fans, and heaters or air conditioners may permeate the environment. What we think of as silence may in fact be quite noisy. People rarely complain about how noisy the ocean is, but waves produce a lot of sound. Leaves on trees make a tremendous sound as they rustle. And if you are in a sensory deprivation chamber, the sound of your heartbeat and your breathing can seem very loud. So noise is not an obstacle to meditation—it is something you make use of. There is never complete silence as long as you are alive to hear, because the rush of blood flowing through your body hums in your ears.

Sound is a wonderful medium of expression and exploration in meditation. You may want to explore some of the sounds that have been used for thousands of years as tools of thought.

Meditation sounds, or mantras, often resemble the sounds people make when they sigh or exclaim in surprise, wonder, awe, and pleasure: Ahh! Ooooh! Eeeeeee! Mmmmmm. . . . These sounds are often soothing and awakening at the same time.

Make a list of all the yawning, sighing-with-relief, exclamation, and orgasm sounds you can think of. Hum them a bit and notice how they feel in your body. Do this now.

Hoo. Whew. Aiee. Oy. Oooooh.

What sounds do you associate with relief?

What sounds do you associate with surprise?

What sounds do you associate with wonder?

What sounds do you associate with delight?

What sounds do you associate with orgasm?

What sounds do you associate with joy?

What sounds do you associate with peacefulness?

Make your own list of favorites right now, before going further with sound. Survey the sounds you sometimes make naturally. What are your favorite sounds? Become intimate with the sounds you love. This will be your foundation for the explorations with sound on the following pages.

You could also set yourself the task of noticing the sounds other people make. As you go to work, watch TV, see movies, talk to friends, play with kids, what sounds do you hear? Comic books often have wonderfully descriptive action sounds—kerPOW!

EXPLORE THE VOWELS OF YOUR MOTHER TONGUE

TIME: 20 minutes.

WHERE: You need uninterrupted conditions for this.

On *Sesame Street* (an educational TV show for children), one of the puppets sometimes walks out waving a sign that says, "This portion of the show is brought to you by the Letter E." Mantras are self-generated sounds that can be used in meditation, and all mantras are brought to you by the Letters of the Alphabet.

One approach to exploring the use of sound in meditation is to relearn the alphabet. This time around you are concerned not with how to write and say the letters, but with recognizing how the sounds resonate in your body. You may have done this once upon a time, when you were learning to speak. Recently I visited a friend who has a two-year-old daughter, Sabrina. The little girl was trotting around the room singing vowel sounds: "Ah—Eeeee—Ah—Eeeee—Ohhhhh—Eeeee." She was clearly delighted by the sounds themselves, and I was too. It was beautiful. She kept improvising and playing with the sound quality of words she was learning: "mmmmMmmmmmOmmmmeeeee" (Mommy).

What Sabrina was doing was playing with the mantric quality of speech, meaning the vibration itself and how it feels in the human body. The main difference between her playing and your meditating with a mantra is that in meditation, you let the mantra fade away and then follow it into the silence, whereas Sabrina was much more interested in dancing with the sound. One thing I learned from her that day was how much OM there is in MOM and MOMMY, something I'd never realized before. OM, as you may know, is one of the great mantras used in yoga and all the Himalayan meditation traditions, including the Tibetan.

In meditation, one tool or technique you can use is listening to the sounds of the alphabet in a special way. Basically, you think a vowel or syllable and let your attention synchronize with its rhythms; then you listen to it fade away. The sound gives you something to focus on that is pleasing in the way that music is pleasing, making you more aware of the silence that comes afterward. In this way, you learn to be alert to emptiness and silence.

Sound is handy for setting up a condition of "delicious underloading of the senses" that is so enjoyable in meditation. You can hum or think a sound at any level, then sit back as it fades. The next few paragraphs show you how to do that. Letting a sound remind you of silence is one of those things that's easier done than said.

Quietly and leisurely, say the vowels and let yourself become comfortable with them. You use them constantly in speaking and thinking, but take a moment to get used to them in a meditative mood. Explore various ways of saying and thinking the vowel sounds. Notice that you can think a sound, then listen, and there is a feeling of the sound's echo or afterglow.

Identify the vowel sounds you feel best with and make a note of them, for you will use those sounds to construct your mantras. When you think in words, the sound is there but you usually are not listening to it; you are aware of the meaning of the words. In mantra meditation, you use the ability to think in words and the auditory sensory pathway as a focus for attention.

As with listening to music, feeling subtle sensations and vibrations in the body has a strong kinesthetic component.

Technique

1. Speak, sing, or hum any vowel sound in any language you know, perhaps your mother tongue if you are bilingual.

2. If you find yourself singing, you can also hold on one note and then glide through the vowels, noticing which ones give you the most pleasure.

   If you are saying the vowels, just notice which ones you feel attracted to or enjoy the most.

3. Glide around, because the vowels are mixed anyway—in English, for example, a, e, and i all have the "eee" sound. Make up variations of the vowel sounds. Play with them as a child would. Take an "oh"

sound and let it shift to "ou" as in "you." Take the "ay" sound and notice how it feels to say "ah."

Notice the way you shape your lips and where you position your tongue.

4. *Select one of the vowels and hum it, with the lips closed, to sense the vibration in your mouth. Do this for several minutes.*

5. *Then say it quietly, barely mouthing the sound.*

6. *Listen inside yourself as the sound shifts from being something you make in your throat and mouth to a sound that is echoing inside you.*

7. *Take the attitude of not caring whether the sound is there or not, and simply pay attention to your bodily feelings.*

Do this for five minutes or so.

This exercise will help you appreciate poetry as well as vocal music, because poets and singers use many exquisite techniques in placing and shaping vowels. The more you explore vowels in meditation, the more your body will open to take pleasure in poetry and music.

CHANT THE VOWELS

TIME: 1 minute to 5 minutes.

WHERE: Anywhere you don't mind being heard.

Chant the vowels of any language you know, in any order. Have an attitude of curious exploration and simple pleasure. It helps to give yourself permission to feel childlike and mischievous.

After you get some vowels going, begin to pay attention to the roundness of the sounds, and to the movement in your mouth as you shape the sounds. It's fun.

Each vowel resonates in a different place in your skull and in your body.

Stay with one pitch and slide through the vowels.

Then let the tone change, like a song, and play with going up and down.

If you are playful, you will probably make up your own variations. Experiment with chanting softly, then really belting it out.

Add any consonants you like. For example, if you are chanting "Ah," notice what happens if you add *y* to get a "Yah" sound. If you are chanting *e* sounds or *i* sounds, feel what happens when you add *mmmm* or *n*.

In English, *-ing* is added to many verbs to indicate ongoing action. Chant-ing, breath-ing, sing-ing, play-ing. Check out what happens to your chant when you add the "ing" sound to any vowel.

Many people find that chanting the vowels clears the head in just a minute. It is refreshing, relaxing, and energizing. Letting the voice relax helps make ordinary speaking seem more pleasurable.

◎ Variations

Let's say you have found a vowel combination you particularly enjoy, such as AH-EE.

Take the time to find the consonants that really spice up the sound for you.

For example, with AH-EE, if you add sh at the beginning, an n and a t sound, you have Shanti, the Sanskrit word for peace.

Shanti is pronounced SHAN-TEE.

Sanskrit is onomatopoeic: it sounds like what it means. Chant SHANTI for ten minutes and see how you feel. This works both ways; if you find a vowel combination that seems to produce a certain effect in your body, you are in a way making up your own Sanskrit. It is good for everyone who uses spoken language to have a feeling for how sound resonates in the body.

Another sound with AH-EE is Shakti, which is the female aspect of divinity. A woman I know loves to chant Shiva-Shakti, meaning the union of male and female divinity. Shiva is pronounced SHEE-VAH and Shakti is pronounced SHAK-TEE.

In the worldview that Sanskrit emerged from, everything is divine, including every sound of every letter, including the ones you use all the time without thinking about it.

At different times of the day, or when you are in different moods, different sounds may call you.

> *Ma, the word for mother in Sanskrit, is part of many chants and mantras. You can make up combinations of sounds with Ma:* MA EEEEE MA. MA-YA.
>
> *Ram is a wonderful, masculine, radiantly solar sound, often said as Rama or Ra-Ma. So the sound has male and female integrated in it. It is used in many chants and mantras.*
>
> *Yah is a fantastic sound. The Germans use it for Yes; vocalists and back-up singers use it as a generally affirming filler sound, as in "Yeah, yeah, yeah." It combines with everything.*

LISTEN TO SILENCE

TIME: Half an hour.

WHEN: At four in the morning, or in nature (for example, in the mountains), or in a silent cathedral.

Silence has a music to it. You can sometimes hear it when you are in a silent area of nature. Sometimes you can hear it in the still time several hours before dawn, even in an urban area.

Do a breathing awareness technique or any other meditation to get in.

Then simply listen. Put your attention into your ears, very gently. In the silence, the ears seem to open up and become intensely receptive.

The silence can seem like a hum, a vibration, a pure clear emptiness that is somehow harmonious, or simply vast.

People describe it as sweet, clarifying, musical, comforting, slightly terrifying, electrifying, and enlightening.

Sometimes it's like a prolonged "ing" sound, or high-pitched "eee" sounds, or a hiss. (The sound is different from tinnitus, which is a ringing in the ears caused by nerve damage or high blood pressure.)

LISTEN TO THE MOST BEAUTIFUL MUSIC IN THE WORLD

TIME: 10 to 30 minutes.

Scout out the most beautiful music available to you. You can select pieces you already love, or you could make a project of asking everyone you know, "What is the most beautiful music you have ever heard?" Include in your hunt the resources available in your community: concerts, recitals, choirs, temple services, the records and tapes in libraries.

Then arrange to be able to listen to this music, every day for a week if you can. If you have access to a sound system, get enough music for ten minutes to half an hour a day for a week. The ideal would be to have an appointment with yourself to listen every day, at the same time of day if possible, and to continue for about seven days. Do what you can. If you do not have a sound system, maybe you know someone who has a good one and a collection of music, and you could go there.

If you are in a room with a stereo, sit in a comfortable chair in the sweet spot, if you can. Or sit between the speakers. Arrange not to be disturbed, and make a commitment to stay with the exercise, to stay attentive and with your feelings, no matter what happens. Open your ears and heart to the music and let yourself melt.

As you listen, give over with your entire being to the movement of the music. Surrender to the rhythm. Give your body to the melody and the pulse. Let the music carry you away.

Listen at moderate volume part of the time. Then listen at low volume, then at extremely low volume for one or two minutes. Then sit and simply listen to the silence for about three minutes.

Sit upright and fairly erect the whole time you are listening. If you want to, check in with your breathing as you listen, but mostly, let the music be your meditation.

You could use classical music of any kind, chanting, jazz, Brazilian, or anything else that is to your taste. But see if you can explore new realms.

In doing this simple exercise, you will develop good habits that will carry over into your other meditations. You will also work through some of the obstacles you might encounter in meditation. Because you are just listening to music, you are less likely to try to resist thoughts or emotions; the music will just carry you. You also will give yourself a chance to get used to sitting in a chair being in rapture for an appointed time.

This is an excellent way to begin meditation, and you can do it for a week, a month, a year, a lifetime. The total attentiveness during, and the silence after, makes it meditative.

AH HUM MEDITATION

TIME: 5 to 10 minutes.

1. Sit upright in a comfortable position. It is preferable to have back support and for the feet to be flat on the floor.

2. Let the eyes rest while looking ahead and slightly downward. Then let the gaze expand. Allow your peripheral vision to open up to perceive the space to the left and right and above and below. When your eyes feel like it, allow them to close, and for a few moments continue to appreciate the sense of space around you. Resonance takes place in space, as when you are singing in the shower.

3. Remember a time when you said Hmmmm, or call up the experience of saying Hmmmm to yourself in a natural way, so that you know this is a sound originating from within yourself. Play with the sound a little, and listen with your body for where it resonates and where you would like it to resonate.

4. Then add one or more of the vowels, *a, e, i, o, u,* to the middle. Ham, heem, hiem, hom, hoom, hum. Explore which of these appeals to you the most.

   Give primacy to discovering which of the sounds or combinations pleasure you. There will be a sense of charm, or pleasure. The choice is the same as when you select certain pieces of music to play. All beings know what music they like. Wolves and whales know what sounds they want to sing. Feel free to follow your instincts. As you play with sounds, you will start to get familiar with a sense of guidance from within your own body. It is very simple, just the sense of pleasure or comfort or excitement of the sounds. Sounds can be relaxing and exciting at the same time.

5. Select any two or three of these sounds (such as ee-ah-um) that strike your fancy and say them to yourself quietly for a minute. End with the . . . mmmm sound, but begin with anything you like.

6. Continue saying the sounds softly, listening to the rhythm and music of the vowels. Let yourself feel the resonance of the humming in your body.

7. Allow the outward sound to fade away as you continue to listen to it inwardly. Simply intend that the sound continue, but do not put any effort into it. Be willing for it to continue or not. If it continues, you enjoy the quiet vibration of the sounds; if not, enjoy the silence.

   The effort in this step is less than the effort of moving your eyes to read this page. It is a simple intention that the mantra, or the resonance of it, or the hum of it, continue. Then you simply listen to the mantra, or to the way it changes, or to the absence of the mantra. It's okay for the mantra to go away. At that point, do what you want; do you want to listen to the absence of the mantra, perhaps a sense of inner quiet, or do you want to listen to the mantra some more?

8. Let any part of the sounds expand or contract—that is, take a longer or a shorter time phrase. If your sound is am-ah-hum, then the central "ah" could go on and on at times, as if you will never get to the "hum." That's fine. It's also okay if you think the mantra once at the beginning of the meditation, then don't think it again for five minutes. Just pay attention to the space between sounds. Be that leisurely. There is no rush to return to the sound, and there is no rush to finish a thought you may be absorbed in.

Continue this way for five minutes. Then check to see that there is no strain anywhere in your body and that you are not furrowing your brow to concentrate. Make sure that you are not trying to block out thoughts or outside noises.

Over a period of days, you can increase your time from five to ten minutes. As long as you feel easy during meditation and great afterward, you can go on for up to twenty minutes—although I would prefer that you take at least a month to reach that level. I don't recommend ever going longer than twenty minutes. Sound meditations are intensely relaxing and awakening, and gradualness is everything. You want to take your time getting used to the intensity of relaxation that this type of meditation can produce.

 Variations

Here are some more sounds you might want to play with:

Am ah hum

Ra mah hum

Mah yah hum

Oh mah nah

Somanah

Sonojah

Hri-yah

If you are more comfortable using something religious, take Jesus' name, the way it is sung in hymns, Jesu. Jay-su. In Spanish, Hey-soos. Or if you are a Rastafarian, Yah is a wonderful sound. Hallelujah and Alleluia are ecstatic sounds. One of the most beautiful sounds in any language may be Allah. Listen to that: "All" and "Ah."

Yahoo is a wonderful mantra.

Sound is a very simple experience. You are built to use sound and do so all the time. Sound meditation is just riding sound into silence. Remember, every experience that arises in you during meditation is actually part of your own experience; it is not unique to meditation. It's just that you are awake while being deeply relaxed. You have these experiences all the time when you are asleep. Every mental picture, every wave of thought, emotion, and sensation is part of your meditation experience. Accept it all. Be like the Statue of Liberty, welcoming all immigrants.

Have a clock or watch nearby so that you tell how long you have meditated.

When the time is up, take a full three minutes to sit there before opening the eyes fully. For two minutes, just be aware that you are going to come out of meditation, and start to move, shift, yawn, stretch, breathe deeply. The last minute, experiment with opening the eyes briefly and then closing them again. Slowly let your awareness expand into the space that you were perceiving before you started meditation.

RA-MA MEDITATION

It can take several weeks to get into the Ra-Ma meditation. Proceed *with infinite leisure*. Do one step until it becomes automatic, then proceed to the next.

In ancient Sanskrit literature, this meditation would be described in one sentence: Meditate on Ra in the area of the top of the mouth; meditate on Ma in the area just behind the genitals. Here is what it looks like as a step-by-step instruction.

1. As you breathe in, notice how delicate the touch of air is as it flows over your sensitive membranes. Everywhere breath flows, molecules of you reach out to meet molecules of the air, sampling and savoring it. Breathe in your normal way; simply pay special attention on the inbreath, and rest on the outbreath.

    Your body is already alert to the blessing of the incoming air, so simply be with that alertness. Join with your body as it rejoices in the gift of life.

    Give yourself a few minutes to fall in love with the inbreath.

2. Then, when it feels natural to do so, let the attention rest in the open space of the mouth. Even with the mouth closed, there is a womb there, an open space capable of generation. It can generate speech and sound. The mouth shimmers with potential, with everything yet unsaid or unsung. Enjoy that empty space between the tongue and the roof of the mouth.

    As you get used to attention resting in the mouth, feel around for where specifically it likes to rest: the top of the tongue? the roof of the mouth? the back of the throat? Give yourself a chance to discover.

    There are in the body many little centers of delight; they are like sofas for attention to rest on—places you can snuggle into, places that attract attention for any reason, places where the sensations are somehow different.

    One of them is in the top of the mouth, the palette, and from there it extends upward into the brain.

3. Another is the area of the body around the genitals. Breathing with awareness, notice where in the vicinity of the genitals your awareness can rest. Is it in the genitals themselves or in the space just behind them? As you continue breathing, allow your attention to be attracted to that subtly delightful area. These may be the same areas that call out to be touched in lovemaking. They may be areas you have not discovered yet. They may be areas that you want to have touched only by breath.

   Remember, meditation is an embrace of everything human, all of yourself, everywhere in your body. You are in the privacy of your own body; no one else knows what you are feeling.

4. Get used to alternating attention between the mouth or palette and the genitals. Take as much time as you want to get used to this: days, weeks, months, years.

   Over time, allow this alternating to go with the breath. Again, this may take time. You have time. Proceed with infinite leisure.

5. Consider the sound "Ahh." Open the mouth slightly and let "Ahhhhhhh" resonate in your mouth.

   Or you could use the sound "Raa." It is the sound the Egyptians used for the sun god. The "rrr" sound adds a little juice. Use whichever you wish.

   Now let the "Ahhh" sound or the "Raaa" sound be internal, something you hear inside, with subvocal speech.

6. Consider the sound "Ma" or "Maaaa." Give yourself time to become intimate with this sound. It is easy for babies to make. It is the primordial sound of the feminine.

   Then rest and enjoy the flow of breath. At each step, ease off and rest in yourself, then proceed. This way, you will not develop the habit of concentrating. You want to let your attention get the feeling of enjoyment and ease at each and every step. You proceed with such leisure that the mind of itself wants to move to the next step.

7. In some moment when you have been enjoying all the above, let attention sway between Ra and Ma, the mouth and the genitals area. Be alert to the vibrations of Ra in the mouth and Ma in the genitals.

8. Explore the alignment of your head. Sometimes leaning forward slightly makes for a more intense experience.

9. Then begin to pause at the end of the inbreath and savor the vibrations.

10. Exhale and pause and attend to the vibrations.

Getting into Attention

PAYING ATTENTION WITH LOVE

Meditation is a lot about attention, all the ins and outs of it. Paying attention is similar to loving—if you love someone, or something, you have attention for her or him or it. It is a delight to pay attention. It's easy.

The word *attention* is etymologically related to *tenderness*. Attention, tender, tend to it.

In the outer world, we pay attention: we are interested, we feel wonder, appreciation, curiosity. When you pay attention to yourself, you use the same attention and let attention be tender. Loving attention is a tender appreciation of your humanity—all the paradoxes and complexities of your incarnation.

Enrich your attention continually. Let yourself learn to love from everything you do: music, art, literature, love relationships, meditation, children, playtime, parties, study. You can learn to love yourself and be tender toward yourself by having friendships with people who are healthy human beings.

MEDITATION IS BEING WITH WHAT YOU LOVE

Meditation techniques are ways of paying attention to life that you never tire of. It's obvious, if you think about it. How else could people

NOTE: Even though I have decades of meditation experience, it would probably take me days to get into this meditation, doing it a few minutes a day. If I did it just the right amount per day, then my body would look forward to doing it. If I overdid it, the meditation would start to feel like work rather than a delight.

I could learn more quickly if someone guided me through it—I'd save a few days. But this is the kind of thing you can learn on your own if you are patient. There are quite a few steps, and you want to approach those steps in such a way that you get intimate with each one and one step naturally flows into the next.

It is not as complicated as learning to sew, or cook, or sing. In meditation you want to learn a thing in the same easy way that you will do it, because meditation is about learning to do almost nothing. You are paying attention, but it feels easier than watching TV or even sleeping. Although this meditation is classical, it is also akin to what some singers learn.

meditate for years? All meditation techniques are derived from ways of paying attention that worked so well, that were so delightful, that someone just fell into them naturally. Meditation is not rocket science. It is surrender to love. What are meditation techniques? Breath, listening to internal music, paying attention to light and to the Light of Awareness, movement itself. Meditation techniques are things you would delight to attend to for years.

The whole idea of a breath meditation is to fall in love with breath. Love is a state of perceiving great value in the beloved. In meditation great value is experienced in the things everyone takes for granted: the air we breathe, space, sound, light, movement, gravity, existence.

Always remember, have it as your touchstone, that meditation is being with that which you love. Your path in meditation will emerge from exploring what it is you love to pay attention to. The skills of attention are the skills of rapport and intimacy with the self.

WHAT DO YOU REALLY LOVE?

What do you really love doing? What images, activities, people, come to mind? What remembered sense impressions do you hear or feel?

It could be anything. You could be in any time of your life past or present, in any country, alone or with someone or many people. Go with whatever pops into your mind right now and let the memory become vivid.

Which of your senses are most active? Which senses bring you the greatest joy? What do your eyes see, your ears hear, your body feel when you are in the midst of that joy? Let yourself become completely immersed in the experience. Take as long as you like.

You could be fly-fishing, playing piano, cuddling, making love, lounging in bed in the morning, driving fast, waterskiing, singing, watching a movie, anything. How do you see the world? How do you perceive colors and sounds? What do you smell? How long do you linger with that smell?

Be in your body and notice how you breathe when you are engaged in that activity. Take a deep breath now, as if you are inside that experience. What does it feel like to breathe? Are you breathing freely? Are you so excited that you are breathing rapidly? Explore.

Go ahead and give over to what the experience has to teach you. Be there inside your body in that activity, attending to your senses and to life.

Sometimes, when you do this exercise you may recall an activity you do alone. At other times, you may recall experiences that have to do with shared attention.

In shared attention you are attending to someone and he or she is paying attention to you in a special way. In doing the exercise you are internalizing that quality of attention you love, taking it inside

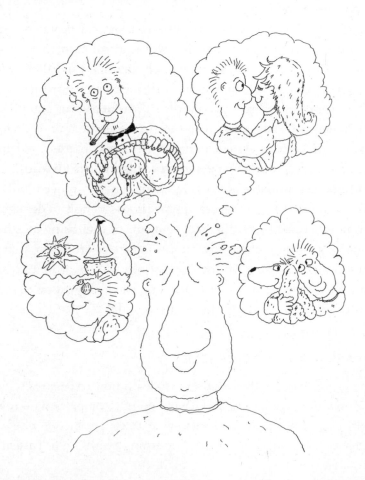

yourself, memorizing the way of it. This could be another person or an animal. Animals can be amazingly attentive and give unconditional love.

Other experiences may be solitary but may not feel so because you are being with yourself.

As you enter the experience of that activity, notice how you are paying attention. What quality of alertness do you have? Are you vigilantly alert or languidly aware, or somewhere in between?

Reentering your memories of your favorite times will teach you about the qualities of attention you love and crave.

Reminder: Pause and take a few breaths as you read.

Always be alert to the qualities of attention you love. Cultivate them in yourself and others.

You can do this exercise a few minutes a day for years and never come to the end of it. Over time you will learn to enjoy the sense of inquiry also, the process of asking yourself questions and then receiving answers in whatever language the body speaks in the moment.

When you recall an experience, it is real as far as your brain is concerned. When you call up an experience in the context of meditation, you give your nervous system permission to remap itself and make more connections. Your nervous system wants to have all learning, all its best resources available at every moment. The brain needs only the slightest permission to do this remapping. It knows how to defragment itself, how to weave all the disparate elements of your being together.

Some people think of meditation as subtractive attention, that you get there by deleting everything interesting. This is an option—the hermit cave dweller's path—but there is no particular reason to seek it out if you live in the world. So let your colors fly.

COMPASSION FOR YOURSELF

One of your tasks with attention is to learn how to be good to yourself. Compassion starts at home. If you are not compassionate toward yourself, how can you be compassionate toward someone else? The word *compassion* is made up of *com-* (meaning "with") plus *passion*. Be with your passion.

If you do not make meditation a healthy place right from the start, it's likely that it never will be. Healthy means you do not repress yourself, brutalize yourself, edit yourself. You want to accept all impulses so that they can join the family, become integrated. Any part that is excluded becomes slightly insane. Good healthy anger that is blocked can then seem like feral rage. But when you accept it and work with it, it becomes the ability to stand up for yourself.

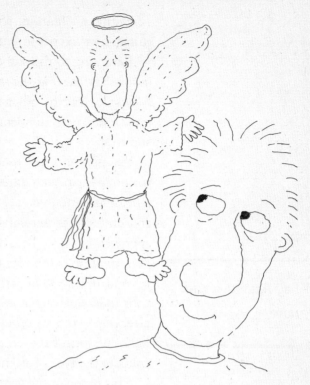

If you do not intentionally cultivate your best attention in your native state, then you will tend to recapitulate the worst attention your kindergarten teacher or parent gave—disapproval, criticism, scrutiny.

When you develop compassion for yourself, you will discover that even the most critical of your inner voices is trying to love you.

GIVING AND RECEIVING LOVE

Attention is a many-splendored thing. In love, in business, and in meditation, you find yourself engaged with many *tones* of attention. Each has its own value and purpose. Each is a different way of relating to the world. You move between these modes naturally, all the time, and you always have.

When you meditate, you exercise the full range of attention. What I am calling the different tones of attention are the parts of that range, as individual colors are the parts of a rainbow.

Let's say you are out on a romantic date with a new love. You may find yourself paying attention with: appreciation, admiration, curiosity, wariness, delight, longing, and amusement. Notice that the type of attention changes slightly from moment to moment. You may look across the table at someone and find yourself switching from curiosity to delight, or from wariness to amusement.

During meditation, you may find the same kind of rapid changes going on as you pay attention to yourself.

Returning to the story above, let's say that years later, you are still in love and meet at the same restaurant to celebrate your relationship. As you look at the other, you may feel yourself moving between adoration, tenderness, amusement, respect, compassion, passion, devotion, and trust.

You may also feel yourself receiving these qualities from the other person, perhaps in a different order. Or you may feel a hankering for a type of attention you are not getting. Maybe you crave understanding and enthusiastic reassurance, and instead you are aware of receiving approval.

Pay Attention with Love

Attention is the very texture of a relationship. Each of the tones is a wonderful world of perception and can be explored endlessly. Part of your individual signature, your personality, is the sequence of types of attention you give other people and the speed at which you switch back and forth between them. Other people, when they think of you, think of the type of attention you give and ask for.

This is one of the ways you can learn how to pay attention to yourself in meditation. You can draw on the way you feel when you are being loved and listened to by an old friend, even one who has died or moved away. As you practice paying loving attention to all the material of the self presented to you in meditation, you are learning to love other people as well.

If you want to give love a chance to survive, know intimately the kind of attention you are good at giving, know the attention you crave to receive, and know both how to give and how to receive. Then work to extend your range of both giving and receiving.

This is where meditation comes into play. A simple way of describing meditation is: to take a bath in attention and absorb all its qualities. Even though each of us specializes in giving certain types of attention and feels a shortage of other types, somewhere in our soul we know all types. In meditation, the body frees itself of the restrictions imposed by our everyday activity and renews its contact with the fullness of life.

SETTING ATTENTION FREE

As you explore meditation you will find that you have, not only a set of modes of attention, but also a speed at which you switch among them. In meditation, almost everyone has a tendency to violate his or her speed and tone. But doing so makes meditation difficult, or at least less interesting. Alert yourself not to do this.

If you are watching a presentation at a business meeting, you may find yourself leaning forward with interest or leaning back with detachment. And your attention will tend to shift among various tones. The mix will probably vary depending on the situation, but you will move among tones of attention, as appropriate.

Interest
Suspicion
Skepticism
Pleasure
Enthusiasm

The situation is no different if you are paying attention to your breath during meditation. You might delight in breath one second, be soothed by it the next, fall asleep a few seconds later, and wake up horny half a minute later, wonder what time it is, then realize that you feel extremely well. All this shifting is how life refreshes itself.

People bore themselves out of their skulls by trying to make meditation one monotonous tone. So do the opposite: set yourself completely free in meditation. Let your attention roam the universe with rapacious intent if it is so inclined, and return to your breath again and again as a base.

Meditation is interesting when you are aware of your own needs, all of them, and let them emerge in the meditation to be attended to. There are many ways of experiencing your needs and many levels on which they reside.

Let your needs come to the surface. They will anyway. You will be tempted to call what you hear mental noise, but it is your inner life coming to the fore to be attended to.

SPEEDY MIND

Meditation happens one breath at a time. That's a few seconds; in half a minute you may breathe in and out eight times. During that time you are likely to be conscious of many thoughts, images, and feelings. The human brain works very quickly.

The people who make commercials know this. They have thirty seconds to convince you that you are unsafe, dirty, ugly, tired, or headachy and that you need their product, which is safe and clean and will make you look beautiful, smell alluring, and live forever. An entire world of beauty is evoked. A lot can happen in half a minute.

Meditation experience comes at you just as rapidly. Fortunately, you have watched a lot of commercials in your life, so you can easily handle your meditative experience if you don't resist. Get used to the speed and intensity. In reality, you think and feel just as fast all the time. Not only is it not a problem, it is a profound adaptation to the necessities of life. The brain doesn't slow down during meditation, nor should it.

When you close your eyes to meditate, you have to respond to or accept your experiences second by second. That is why I tend to refer to meditation as a sport rather than a mind skill. It is a mind skill, but what people think of as mind isn't mind. Mind is the entire body. Your whole body is your brain.

As an exercise, consciously watch some commercials. Notice the speed at which the scenes change, how much information is being presented for you to process, and how easily your nerves ride the changes. In commercials, in life, and in meditation, thirty seconds is a long time.

THE COCKTAIL PARTY EXERCISE

EXERCISE: Go to a party and have a conversation.
PURPOSE: Notice the easy flow of attention.

The next time you are at a party and find yourself engrossed in a fascinating conversation with someone, notice how effortlessly you concentrate on the back-and-forth of the communication. You and everyone else there can be involved in a conversation, track new arrivals, scout around, get food and drink, and return to the conversation. All this is effortless fun because Nature has spent about two billion years figuring out how to make a nervous system that can survive.

Another way to notice how easy it is to focus is to read a newspaper or a favorite book in a coffee shop or an airport.

What does this mean for meditation? It means that in meditation you can pay attention to your breathing or other meditation focus with ease even though people may be conversing all around you. It is not at all an "advanced skill" of meditation to be able to focus when there is a lot of background noise, or when other people are whooping it up.

If you are meditating and somewhere within earshot interesting things are going on, you will find your mind going there to check it out. No problem. If you do not resist the process, your attention will of its own accord return to your focus—your breath, or your own thoughts and sensations.

During meditation a kind of internal party is going on at which all your parts—all the areas of your body and brain—are talking to one another. Sometimes you will be completely involved in hearing and seeing and feeling the communication going on, and sometimes you will be immersed in peacefulness, watching all this action as if from a distance.

If ever you feel yourself trying to block out anything while you are meditating—a thought, an external noise, or the movement of your attention toward a conversation—stop, breathe, and even open your eyes. Don't continue.

THE INNER MULTIMEDIA SHOW

As you move through your daily life, you are immersed in a world of external sensory experience: there is an immense variety of sounds, voices, colors, shapes, smells, and tastes to notice. Although your attention is mostly on the outer world, your inner world is vibrating with aliveness, responding to everything that is important to you. Experience is always simultaneously inner and outer. Nothing really changes in this regard when you close your eyes to meditate.

When you close your eyes to meditate, the only difference is that you are not paying as much attention to the outer world. You are paying more attention to the inner world. The inner world can seem like a conversation, a party, a committee, or a family. Much of what is going on there has to do with past and future action in the outer world. The main difference is that during the moments you are meditating, you are not driving a car or working at a job or hanging out with people.

The outer world is there; your inner world is there.

When you are meditating, you are still in a rich world of sensory experience, just as always. You are still seeing things, hearing things, feeling things.

The Play of Inner and Outer Movies

Let's say you and a friend are talking over what movie to see tonight. Neither of you has made up your mind yet—you are just batting the subject back and forth for a couple of minutes. Each of you wants to be happy with the choice, as well as to please the other person.

As you consider your choices, your brain may show you:

- Brief video clips of previews you have seen.
- Still images of movie ads from the newspapers.
- Songs and snatches of dialogue from the previews.
- Phrases selected from reviews you have read, presented either as a voice or as text.
- Auditory replays of comments from people who have seen one of the movies already.
- Images of the actors in other films you have seen.
- Images of the various theaters, inside and out, of the possible lines, crowds, parking problems, and comfort of the seats.
- A remembered smell and taste of a particular theater's popcorn.

Along with these images and sounds, your brain and body will be displaying to you various feelings of evaluation, good, bad, or indifferent, about each image or sound. These feelings may seem abstract to you. Or they may be localized in your gut or your heart; or they may be an overall bodily sensation that you interpret as excitement or aversion, "I really like that actor (or director), but I don't like film noir (or costume dramas)." Reading these bodily feelings may well be a familiar tactic to you as part of your personal intuition, or the process may go on without your noticing it.

This is just part of what is called thinking, and it goes on all the time, whether you are walking down the street, talking, or deciding where to have lunch. It even goes on part of the time when you are asleep, in which case it's called dreaming.

These elements of thinking—all the moving and still mental images, the remembered music and dialogue, the feelings and sensations evaluating the internal multimedia experience—can be combined in thousands of ways. Every human being has her or his own multimedia thinking "signature," a distinctive set of styles for selecting and combining elements. Just as your voice is distinctive, so is your style of displaying mental images, sounds, and feelings.

So when you are in the process of deciding which movie to see tonight, you are making mental movies about what movie to see, watching the mental movies, and then somehow deciding which of your choices to pursue. This is part of what thinking is, and we are all so good at it that we do it all the time without even paying much attention, just as we can walk down a street without having to pay attention to each step we take.

This is also the reason we like movies. They fascinate us because they are like the thought process. Reality does not jump from scene to scene, but our memories and dreams and internal video imagery certainly do. This is thinking, and human beings do a lot of it all the time, including when they are meditating. Write this on your hand: Thoughts are not a problem. Welcome all thoughts.

During meditation you are in the multimedia theater of your mind, Feel-O-Vision, with a great sound system. You can adjust the dials, turn the volume up or down, change seats, play different movies, even make movies. There are many meditation techniques—as many techniques as there are ways of doing things with photography, film, painting, sculpting, and sound. Meditation is the process of paying attention to the details of thought creation. It is also cleaning the lenses and all the equipment; sorting through the archives; tuning up the equipment; making sure all the connectors and plugs are properly connected; making sure the electricity that powers it all is secure.

Meditation is vastly simpler than thinking. You are mostly witnessing thinking, checking in with your inner television screen and stereo, tuning up the equipment, sorting the memories, taking five, resting, enjoying yourself.

Once you have decided how long to meditate and where, you don't have to decide anything else.

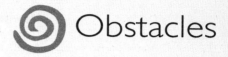 Obstacles

---

**How to Handle Everything in Meditation—
These Are the Rules**

- *THOUGHTS.* Welcome thoughts, even painful thoughts. Thinking is the brain's natural sorting process.

- *EMOTIONS.* Accept the review of emotions. You will feel all the emotions you missed or did not complete during the day, the week, or your lifetime.

- *SENSATIONS.* Welcome the sensations of relaxation and tension release, and get used to them. You will have thousands of kinds of sensations, and most of them will be side effects of relaxation. There is no way to relax for long without the body going into a cycle of releasing built-up tension.

- *NOISE.* Noise is no problem unless you decide to make it a problem (see "How to Make Yourself Miserable in Meditation"). If you can read a newspaper in a restaurant, you can handle external noise while you are meditating.

The Law of Odious Rules

The Law of Odious Rules says: Every meditator has to invent at least one rule that makes meditation difficult if not impossible. For example, because meditation is generally thought of as sitting still, some people make up a Wiggling Is Forbidden rule for themselves. If you can't think of any such rules right now, consult this handy list:

How to Make Yourself Miserable in Meditation

- Sit in uncomfortable postures.
- Meditate longer than you want to or need to.
- Resist thoughts. Demand a blank mind.
- Resist falling asleep.
- Sit in a stuffy room.
- Choose a tradition or meditation that reminds you of the worst aspects of your childhood.
- Don't listen to your inner voices.
- Worry about whether you are being a good meditator.
- Try to achieve enlightenment.
- Suppress your emotions.
- Use a mantra that grates on your nerves.
- Worry about whether your chakras are balanced.
- Resent all noises.
- Wear new, uncomfortable contact lenses while meditating.
- Ban specific types of thoughts, such as sexual thoughts or angry thoughts.

If you are sitting in a group of ten people for a meditation class and the instructor says, "Okay, let's all close our eyes and find something about our breathing to enjoy," maybe five to seven people will do something like that. They will find something to enjoy. One person will sit there sort of perplexed, not knowing where to begin. A couple of people will be sitting there scowling. If you ask one of them what he is doing, he might say, "I was trying to block out noise." Inquiring further, you would find that he was starting to become aware of his breath, then he heard a sound somewhere, then he briefly wondered what the sound was, then he invented an Odious Rule on the spot that he should not hear the sound, then he got angry (or else he recalled an internalized, angry parental voice), then, disgusted, he returned to his breath. This all took place in ten seconds.

This guy is not going to have a happy time in meditation. His critical inner voice will win every time. Not only that, it will get to score a hit on him by proving that he failed at meditation.

You, on the other hand, are not getting expensive coaching on your meditation technique. Think of all the money you are saving! But that means you will have to pay a little attention to these things and go a little more slowly. Be alert to when you are about to make up an Odious Rule, and start making fun of it.

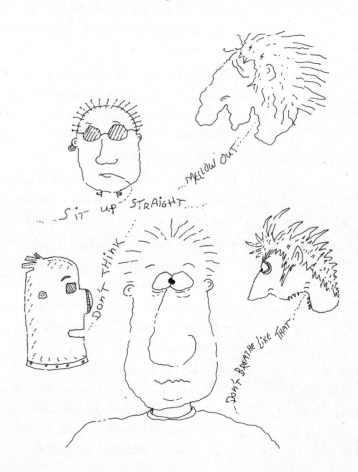

The rules can vary from person to person. For one person it might be "You have to make your mind blank," and for another it might be "You have to believe in the teacher" or "You're not allowed to feel too happy" or "Mood swings must be controlled." Sometimes it is just the voice of the Inner Rebel that must be banned and obliterated with the drone of a mantra.

One way of finding out if you are being run by an Odious Rule is to notice whatever you call "difficult." If you have any feeling of difficulty at any time during meditation, check in with what rules you have made up. When people say meditation is "difficult," often one or more of the following things is going on:

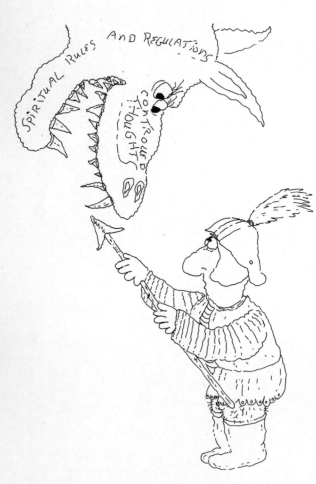

- Many thoughts are coming, and *everyone knows* you aren't supposed to think during meditation.

- Some thoughts flash through very rapidly, and *everyone knows* thoughts should obey the thought speed limit, moving slowly, gracefully, with immense decorum, like a funeral procession.

- Sensations in the body are calling for attention, and *everyone knows* that the body is supposed to be numb during meditation.

- Tension is being released—the body is going into relaxation and by contrast the tense areas show up—and *everyone knows* that tension is supposed to disappear instantly, like kitchen stains do in TV commercials.

- Emotions are welling up and you don't want to feel them. *Everyone knows* you're not allowed to cry during meditation. Or else "unauthorized" emotions are coming up. This is different for everyone.

What you may be encountering here is your internal manual of meditation. It already knows everything there is to know about everything. Its title is "How to Make Yourself Miserable" or "Meditation Made Difficult." As you pay attention in an easy way, you contradict the inner programming about making things difficult.

This tendency to make things difficult is just in our culture. Not everyone has to deal with it right away, but all meditators have to deal with it eventually. If the Made Difficult instruction set comes up and wants to take over your meditation, just make fun of it. Don't get into a struggle with the tendency to make things difficult. It's a tar baby.

When you approach the activity of meditating in a healthy way, you violate all the dysfunctional rules you may have learned along the way: don't feel, don't think, don't wiggle, don't ask questions, don't be angry, don't be sexual, don't doubt, don't be a rebel, don't do it your own way, do it the official way.

What Do I Do About . . .

THOUGHTS

The situation: Much of the time when thoughts come during meditation, you will be completely carried away by them. You will forget you are meditating and be busily planning something or reviewing something you did earlier in the day. This is healthy; it is part of the brain's natural functioning. The brain and nerves do this kind of processing whenever you rest. This goes on all the time when you sleep, particularly when you dream, and it would be unhealthy to try to resist it during meditation.

So try this attitude on: when thoughts come, they come. Take a welcoming attitude, as if birds have just landed on your lawn. Let them peck around. When you become aware that you are thinking, then you have a choice: you can finish the thought or you can return to the breath or whatever your focus is. When you become aware that you are thinking, do not hurry back to the breath and do not feel you were wrong to be thinking.

You are not responsible for the content of your thoughts in meditation. Nor are you responsible for the speed, frequency, color, or tone of voice. You are responsible for thoughts when you act on them, and in meditation you are not acting on thoughts.

Your mind may feel, sound, and look tremendously noisy to you when you are meditating. This is because the brain and nerves are sorting and filtering. The body has to check every "panic button" you pushed during the day, or since the last time you meditated, and see if you really, truly want a state of total bodily emergency declared because your red dress did not come back from the cleaners on time. Part of what we learn from meditation is perspective—to have the

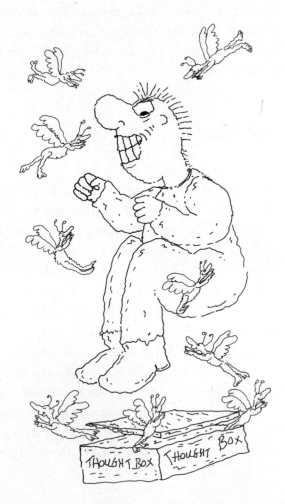

kind of balanced view about today's events that we might get with time, with days or weeks, months or years. There is no way to do this other than by sorting through your everyday experience.

Thoughts do not "appear" out of "somewhere" and take over your brain. Thoughts are already there, and you are quiet enough to hear them or see them. As they emerge from the background noise, attention selects them and begins to sort them out, to extract the lessons from that arena of experience.

Your task is to witness them. There are restless thoughts, planning thoughts, memories of the day, reviews of conversations you want to have, painful memories, good memories, joyous memories.

There are various conditions of relationship with thoughts: being lost in thoughts, becoming aware that you are lost in thoughts, being aware that thoughts are there in the background but still being aware of your breath, a "light cloud" of thoughts, a storm of thoughts.

There are thoughts about thoughts:

> I really shouldn't be thinking this . . .
> I really shouldn't be thinking so much . . .
> Okay. You thoughts, that's enough! Shut up.
> Grrrrrrrr. . . . If it wasn't for these thoughts, I would be peaceful.
> Hey, that's a pretty interesting thought. I think I'll sneak off and play with it a bit.

There are visual thoughts and auditory thoughts. The visual thoughts can be brief images, still photos, or video clips, and they can appear anywhere in your mind's vision field. Auditory thoughts can be stereo or mono, and they can be simulations of various people's voices. There are many different bodily feelings that co-occur with thinking, "gut feelings" that people sometimes call instinct or intuition.

This is only a sampling. There is very little, if anything, in human experience that a meditator does not sift through over the course of months and years of meditation.

So don't worry about controlling or editing your thoughts during meditation.

EMOTIONS

Emotions include joy, sorrow, reverence, hate, and love, to name a few. Over time, you will experience and reexperience almost every human emotion while you are meditating. This is part of the brain's balancing and integrating activity. Your task is to allow the emotions to flow and to breathe with them.

During meditation, every part of your being talks to every other part. One level of this communication is experienced as image and sound, or "thinking." Another level plays through us in the sensations of flow we call "emotion." The word *emotion* is very cleverly constructed: e-motion, just so we don't forget that emotions move.

In meditation, the central attitude should be to welcome the flow and the motion of emotions, and to pay attention whenever and wherever your attention is called. Always give priority to paying tender attention to emotion, and never try to override an emotion using the meditation focus.

You may find yourself feeling things, and finishing feelings, from many years ago. You may find yourself immersed intensely in emotions having to do with today, or yesterday, or tomorrow. Some will have been in suspended animation since a loss or trauma years ago, and now they feel safe enough to emerge.

The nervous system is concerned with building connections, with making your emotional life one seamless tapestry rather than a jumble of fragmented or disjointed experiences. The body wants to have any and all emotions available at a moment's notice, as appropriate, and to be able to express each.

Emotions come up during meditation because you have created a refuge for yourself, a place where you feel safe. You are at home in yourself, so you can cry or get really angry or feel like dying or become blissfully happy. As your body gets used to the refuge, you may find yourself shifting rapidly between very different emotions. You are not going crazy; your brain is just busily getting up-to-date. You may be tempted to try to bring it under control and impose some sort of false equanimity, but don't. Welcome the emotions and simply pay attention.

Many women cry during meditation for the first few months, then feel much lighter and freer. Other people laugh a lot during and after meditation for months after beginning. Usually, day in and day out, the emotional content of your meditation will be whatever you were feeling all day but did not have the time or attention to attend to.

As difficult as this emotional processing seems at times, give yourself the attention. You will feel much freer after meditation. If you have a hard time being tender toward yourself, seek out people who are good at doing what friends do. You can learn from any healthy person how to pay attention to human feeling without blocking it. Cultivate people in your life who are good at emotional expression, and learn to celebrate emotions with the attitude of "the more the merrier." All the explosions of life—anger, tears, laughter—are natural ways for the body to reset its fuses. Whatever feelings you deal with through conversation, dance, sports, music, or art will not be stuck in your body for you to feel while meditating.

If you are stuck, get help: there are psychotherapists, dance therapists, art therapists, and relationship teachers who can help you learn to let emotions flow.

BODILY SENSATIONS

During meditation you will feel a huge variety of sensations in your body, all having to do with the relative level of tension and relaxation you are in at the moment. These sensations change from second to second, and sometimes, paying attention to them is the best thing to do. Usually your attention will be called by a set of sensations. You can trust this calling, for it is the body's way of saying it needs a little help. When you place your attention in any area of the body, the circulation immediately increases there. There is more to this than just increased blood flow, however; attention itself is healing.

In your evening meditations, you may sometimes find your body doing a sort of fast-forward rapid replay of the day's sensations. This roller-coaster adventure can be confusing to beginners, but it is just a side effect of relaxation. Your body is freeing itself up by stripping away the anxiety correlated with performance.

There is often a layer of sensation underneath emotional experience. After the most intense part of the feeling has passed, you can shift to paying attention to the bodily sensations beneath the emotions. You may find sensations in your belly, pelvis, chest area (the "heart"), and throat. These sensations may be electric, clammy, creepy, disgusting, joyous, cold, warm, or fearful. You can also shift your attention to the bodily sensations if you find yourself in a recurrent series of images or voices.

These sensations are what people often refer to as "gut feelings," and they can be very intricate and sophisticated. Anytime you are deeply relaxed, your body, nervous system, and brain, acting in concert, go into a mode of "sorting gut feelings." The body is attempting to learn from past experience and come to an accurate assessment of the present. Having clear and accurate gut feelings is one of the great joys of life, and one of the greatest gifts of meditation.

One reason for meditating in brief sessions, such as five to ten minutes, is so you can get used to the sensations that go with relaxation. There is a lot to learn about moving through your world with your sensors open. The more gradually you engage in this, the better.

If you meditate more than about twenty minutes, too much relaxation can carry over into your daily activity, and you are probably not used to having such a rich experience of your body. Your skin may feel too sensitive to be out among crowds, for example. If you build up very gradually, you will be able to tell what amount of meditation is just right for you.

What About Painful Sensations?

As you begin to rest and relax in meditation, you may become aware of underlying pain or discomfort, such as:

- Sore muscles from physical labor or exercise.
- Lower-back or neck pain from postural problems.
- Tension in various parts of the body: the jaw, shoulders, eyes, belly.
- Pain in the nerves from work or long hours.
- Stiffness from not moving around enough.
- Fatigue from post-flu syndrome.

- Pins-and-needles sensations from restoring blood flow to tensed muscles.

Don't dismay. The paradox is, as you settle into meditation, places in your body that have been habitually tight will start to soften and let go and will feel uncomfortable. When an area has been tensed and then relaxes, there is a period of discomfort as balance is restored.

This is why it is important to make yourself as comfortable as possible when you meditate, so you can tolerate the discomfort that can accompany getting into body awareness. Therefore, let yourself shift around or stretch in any way when you are in meditation. Let the Stillness in Motion, Slump, and Tense to Relax exercises help you here.

If you work long hours and then meditate in the evening, it could well be that most of your sensations are painful. Usually these are tiny pains: crinkly sensations in the skin, on the face, around the eyes, or all over the body; prickly feelings in the heart and belly. They can go on and on, for ten minutes or twenty minutes, the entire meditation. These sensations are often accompanied by images and recalled conversations, and they come with emotional content. You will become well acquainted with this process if you work hard and then meditate.

It is a brave decision to meditate after work when you are tired and stressed! It takes courage to face the pain of fatigue so directly. The reward can be that in half an hour you emerge from meditation feeling renewed, and when you eat dinner even the simplest food tastes delicious. Many people report feeling better all evening after meditating, and then they sleep better because they are already relaxed.

If you are willing to pay attention, and if you stay right there breathing with the painful sensations, they will change gradually, with seemingly infinite slowness. But they will change. The wonder of meditation, and the wonder of the human body, is that you can feel peaceful while you are sitting there feeling your nerves heal, even if they are really irritated. As you learn to trust this process, you will get better at letting the pain pass through you. But this phenomenon is one of the main reasons people quit meditating: they just don't want to sit through the agitation and uncomfortable sensations.

Some people live with pain that is always there, either from injury or disease or because they do not like being in a human body. Although it is natural to want to flee from such pain, people in these situations have reported great benefit from learning to enter the pain and stay there with it.

If you ever find yourself in continual pain, consider attending to it for five minutes every hour. When you do this, you may find your body relaxing into the pain, letting go of the muscular tensions it was using to try to block the pain. This muscular tension is often more uncomfortable than the actual pain.

A surgery patient told me recently of lying in the hospital recovering from an appendicitis operation. The pain was so intense, she said, that her entire body recoiled from it at every movement she made. Yet she hated the way the drugs made her feel. So, with no other good choices, she decided to put her attention right into the pain and feel it. After a while she was able to merge with it and take it. The pain was still there, but she was not doing anything to try to protect herself from it. As she accomplished this, she found her entire body relaxing, letting go of the constrictions it had been doing to try to defend itself against the pain. To her surprise, she felt that the pain of the surgery and of the infection that necessitated the surgery was not as intense as the pain of her own aversion response. Then she discovered that because she was relaxed, she could get up and move slowly about.

You'll have to explore to see what meditation focus is a good support for you to stay there and tolerate whatever sensations of pain you are experiencing. It may be a breath technique, a mantra, or a kinesthetic awareness practice. The pain itself is the main focus, and simple attention the main healer. But sometimes a supporting rhythm, whether of the breath or a sound, is wonderful.

NOTE: Meditation may have made you aware of something that needs medical attention. If so, go get it checked out.

Pain is a calling. It is the body's way of telling you to pay attention. Nothing could be easier, on the level of effort, than to attend to painful sensations when you are meditating. It takes no *effort* to pay attention to the sensations; it takes *willingness* to suffer through the sensations so that your body can heal more quickly.

The Ahhh . . . And the Ouch of Meditation

1. *Ahhhhhh. Physical relaxation.*

2. *Ouch. Reliving tension as you release it. Mental review of what you are tense about as you release the physical tension.*

3. *Ah and Ouch. The sensations that go with deep physical relaxation are sweet and painful at the same time, similar to sitting down or lying down when you are really fatigued. Attending to and feeling into your frayed nerves hurts at the same time it is kind of blissful.*

4. *Oh, No! Suddenly remembering things you forgot to do or realizing that you blew it. Usually there are things you forgot, or ways you could have done something better. Usually this is about small, daily things. Once in awhile it is about something on a larger scale, such as, OHMYGOD, I have been forgetting to enjoy my own life for like the last ten years.*

5. *Grrrr. Anger comes up, whatever you didn't have a chance to feel through or express during the day.*

6. *Boo Hoo. Tears of relief or grief, as the heart opens up to feel. Many times women cry during meditation without knowing why specifically. No particular incident in mind, just a feeling of catharsis. Sometimes there are no tears, just a sinking down into sorrow.*

7. *Ommmmm. There are almost always a few moments of pure repose, very fleeting, but very refreshing. The words Om and home are related somehow. Om is being at home in your body and soul.*

8. *Zzzzzz. Sleep. Usually there are a few moments of sleep.*

9. *Hmmm. After being relaxed for awhile, a sense of reflection about your own life, a sense of wonder, a larger perspective, emerges.*

10. *Wow. As you get used to relaxation, your senses unfold and bring you news of the universe, new perceptions.*

11. *Whew. What a relief.*

12. *Ah Ha! Surprise insights and mini-revelations. I see how to do that!*

13. *Har Har Har. Humor about yourself and life.*

14. *Yahoo. Excitement about what you are going to do after meditating.*

NOISE

Go placidly amid the noise of your mind and the noise in the street, and remember that your brain evolved to deal with it.

Whenever you encounter an experience in meditation that you don't know how to handle, make up a way to handle it gracefully or give up on meditation for the moment. Just don't invent an Odious Rule. Let's take noise as an example. Perhaps you are meditating and you can't stop listening to an interesting conversation in the next room. Or you find yourself listening to sounds you can't identify, and you sit there wondering, trying to visualize what they are. Or a door slams down the hall and you are jarred from feeling peaceful. How do you deal with these situations?

If you are being informal with yourself, then you will deal with the distraction just as you would when reading a novel or magazine. Your attention will flicker over to the outside sounds, assess whether they are life-threatening, then return to your breath or whatever your meditation focus is. Almost anyone can read a novel in an airport or a newspaper in a café with no problem. People do not furrow their brows while reading their favorite escape fiction. A more common challenge for them is remembering to check the time. People can even stand on a busy sidewalk and view a TV news broadcast in a store window. If you watch people concentrating in this way, you will see that they do not strain with concentration. They just watch. If you observe athletes during a game, you'll notice that they tend to have wide-open, almost blank faces. They are concentrating with an open focus. People do this naturally when they are just being themselves. If you are meditating and are this natural, people will think you are an expert. But it is really much easier and simpler *not* to tie yourself up in knots in the first place.

Many times when traveling and staying at people's homes, I have walked out of a room after meditating and the other people have said, "Sorry about the noise while you were meditating," and I have said, "What noise?" This is not a feat of expert meditation. A six-year-old with a comic book can do the same thing. Watching thoughts and perceptions condense out of the dancing chemicals in the brain is just as interesting as reading comic books.

The Odious Rule way would be to resent the outside sounds. Then you can quit meditating and blame the outside world for not shutting up, or you can continue meditating but cultivate anger. This gives you a justification to storm out of the room and scream at people, "Will you hold it down to a dull roar! I'm *trying* to meditate!"

Most people, left to their own devices, will start to resist hearing outside sounds. This is the problem with approaching meditation formally, instead of letting it be as natural as reading a novel. This is the way in which people "doing a technique" are separated from their natural, instinctive way of doing things. They may start to get irritated by the sound, then will try to concentrate. Right here, the meditation is corrupted and you may as well quit.

Some people get irritated at Life or The City and think that other people being alive is an obstacle to meditation. Thus the desire develops to move to a quiet place. But then, nature is very noisy. I live near a bird refuge and the birds make a racket at dawn, singing and chirping away. The blue herons make a weird screeching sound when they glide overhead at dusk. A person could really resent all those noises!

By following the principle of always doing the simplest thing, the well-trained meditator will just let attention stay on the outside noise until it is no longer interesting, then return to breath—because it is more interesting.

During my training to be a meditation teacher, at one point I lived in a hotel on Majorca in winter. It was 1971 or so. The Transcendental Meditation movement liked to rent hotels out of season because we got such great deals. Because it was the off-season, though, construction was going on all over town—lots of jackhammers and dynamiting early in the morning right next to my hotel. I could have made this a problem. But I was having too good a time to do that. I was dynamiting the obstacles inside my psyche, so what was going on in the outer world was a perfect metaphor. A nervous system knows how to deal with noise; you just have to let it do its thing.

All this is another example of how practicing a "technique" can make you stupid. Leave a person alone to read a newspaper in a nice coffee shop in the afternoon, and the person sits there gratefully enjoying the experience. No one sits in Starbucks on a busy street thinking, "If only there were no traffic, if only no one moved or made a sound, then I could enjoy my cup of coffee."

When meditators do not let meditation be simple, what they are practicing is not meditation but resentment—the Resentment technique. If you know any people like this, watch out! Sooner or later their resentment will want to find a two-legged target.

SLEEPINESS

Sleep is to be welcomed. It is wonderful if you fall asleep during meditation. Most busy people have a sleep debt of several dozen hours. When you pay it off, you will feel a lot better; you'll feel younger and lighter. When you are meditating, you sometimes get so relaxed that you will fall asleep sitting up in your chair.

If you nod off, fine. When you wake up, do not try to return to the focus for a while. Just sit there for a minute and let your brain wake up. You will know when you are awake again. Then continue meditating.

Have a blanket and pillow nearby so you can lie down and sleep.

There will be times when taking a nap is by far the most profound meditation you can do.

URGENCY

Sometimes when you sit to meditate you will be inundated with a sense of urgency about doing this and that. Suddenly you'll think of all the things you have to do. This is not a problem—just witness the urgency. For the time being, that feeling itself is your focus. The urgency may be unpleasant, but hang in there; it is very worthwhile to permeate urgent feelings with attention.

On the first level, the urgency is associated with specific tasks left undone or specific topics about which you are concerned. On the next level, the urgency is a feeling in your body, maybe an adrenaline rush in your belly. And farther on in, the urgency is a buzzing in your nerves.

Learn to track these levels; it will be a good thing for you.

Always remember, when this sense of urgency comes up, it's because you have a life and have things to do. The feeling of wanting to do things is to be cherished. What's going on is that your brain is combining relaxation and attentiveness with the electricity of urgency. If you stay with it, you'll emerge balanced. It's a good use of ten or twenty minutes to filter the anxiety out of your action plan.

Everyone who is engaged with the world has feelings of urgency about things that need to be done *now*. There will be times during meditation when you'll find yourself shifting from being deeply relaxed to feeling urgency zap through your body like lightning. This is not a problem—just witness the urgency. Urgency is a sense of need, and you are available to your own feelings of need. Feeling your urgency in meditation is perfect, because the urgent feelings really need to be combined with inner resources, with calm inner strength, and this is what happens in meditation. If you do this, you will find that you emerge from meditation energized. Some or most of the urgency will have been transformed into excitement and real energy, and there will be less anxiety.

The urgency is not your meditation technique; your technique is to pay tender attention to the urgency as a set of feelings in your body. The urgency probably has a set of pictures with it, pictures of tasks you need to do. The only thing to watch out for is not letting the urgency push your technique.

Many people feel that they have failed to meditate properly when feelings of urgency come up, and acting on this misinformation, they try to *do* something. They may try to do one of two things, either of which will immediately sabotage their meditation. They:

1. Try to suppress the urgency in order to calm down.
2. Urgently try to "get into" meditation. They may be tempted to rush into breath to escape from the tension.

Either or both of these will corrupt the simplicity of attention and will make meditation seem like work. What you do is simply let the urgent feelings call your attention, and continue to pay attention as the highly charged thoughts roll through your mind. This usually feels like suffering. So stay with the urgent/anxious/excited feelings until you have matched rhythm with them and there is no suppression in your attitude. Then to your surprise you will find yourself slipping into meditation. This is easier done than said. I had to use all these words to describe something that in practice you can do in a few seconds.

One day a man by the name of Norm came over for a meditation session. He mentioned at the beginning that he was always "aware of time." He looked at his watch a lot and seemed to want to move fast. He had an attitude of "Let's hurry up and meditate." He said he had tried to meditate many times but couldn't "slow his mind down" enough to succeed.

I listened to Norm talk about his relationship with time for a while. Then, because he was a physicist, I asked him, "What . . . is . . . time?" He closed his eyes and didn't want to open them for almost half an hour. He was in a deep reverie, experiencing his own body as a wave in the spacetime continuum. Afterwards, he said he did not feel anxious about time, as he did before, but excited by being able to play in the fields of time. Norm had told me that his work involved using supercomputers to make animated imagery of physics equations, so I figured he would have a lot of fantastic mental imagery, and he did.

This was a breakthrough for Norm, and you will have your own at some point when you are meditating and the sense of urgency arises in you. Urgency is the pulse beat of your own life, and ultimately the dynamic impulse of life itself, which is always wanting to move on. This is not an obstacle to meditation; rather, it is a great ally.

MOODS

If you are moody, meditate anyway. Moods are a bit vaguer than emotions. By "moody" I mean:

Irritable
Bored

Restless

Lonely

Ornery

Horny

Mischievous

Cheerful

Chipper

Sassy

Playful

Amused

Defiant

Creative

Rebellious

Dreamy

You usually can't quite put your finger on the discrete emotion, but you know something's going on. A mood may be associated with a vague feeling all over your body, and you may not even want to pay attention to the mood—you may want to jump out of your skin, or lose yourself in watching TV or some such thing.

Whatever mood you are in, angry or tired or peaceful or excited, you can meditate. All this variety of emotional tones just makes meditation more interesting; it allows you to experience your body in different states. When you find yourself in each mood, that is your opportunity to be with it. Attention is magic. Your attention is called; simply be there while the sensations, emotions, voices, and images last.

While meditating, you may notice very quick movement among your moods, from one to another. Or the movement may not seem quick enough. Breathe with each mood as it comes and as it goes, and let it have a home in your meditation.

Sometimes an entire meditation will be spent processing a mood, soaking in it. Then when you emerge from meditation, to your total surprise, you find you have finished it and feel completely different, as if a weight has been lifted off you.

Welcome your real self. That's what honesty means. Restfulness sometimes means you are resting in your own bad self—from the beginning. You do not have to be an impostor, taking on a false attitude of piety.

Train yourself to welcome "negative experiences." *I'm lonely, bored, horny, angry, tired, irritable, worried about money, hungry, lost, depressed. I don't wanna meditate.* Bring 'em on. You do not have to change any of these moods in order to meditate. These are the gateways into meditation. Your everyday, real life is your work sheet, your material. Your longings, the unfinished places in you, your needs for energy and attention and love, these are the motivators for meditation. You can meditate as a rebel, as a trickster, as a grump.

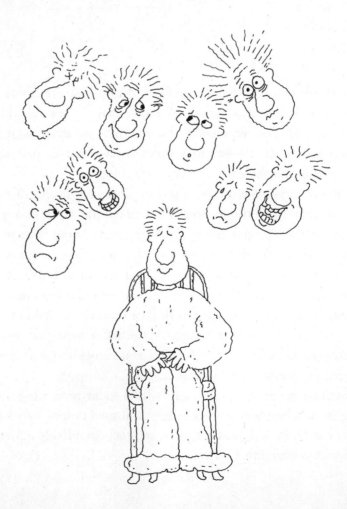

RESTLESSNESS

Welcome your impulses to move. If you feel restless before meditating, you may want to learn a stretch routine or walk for half an hour. Showers help.

Once you start meditating, welcome the restlessness and find out what it wants. Never try to "suppress" restlessness in meditation. If you don't want to do anything beforehand to minimize it, then witness it and ride it; you will learn a lot.

In meditation you do not make yourself sit still. You only sit relatively still, as you would when listening to music or reading a book. When you are reading, you don't have to tell yourself, "Sit still, sit still," as if you were a dog. You don't even think about it. So let yourself stretch, sigh, or scratch. Even when you are in deep meditation, your breath is flowing and your heart is beating. So why get into a struggle with life about movement? If you welcome movement, you will experience more stillness in meditation.

WILD, POLITICALLY INCORRECT IMPULSES

Externally, meditation appears politically correct because no one can see what you are thinking.

Internally, meditation is Wild Time—you cut loose, let your hair down, party, think any outrageous thought that crosses your mind without bothering to edit it. You don't have to go out of your way to think something outrageous, but you don't have to maintain a guard against thinking it either. That would be too much work. You don't need to edit during meditation because you aren't going to act on the thoughts. So why bother to edit? Meditation time is like when you dream at night.

During the day, we are all constrained in many ways. We conform our behavior to whatever situation we find ourselves in. This is good. This is called civilization. It is good that you didn't murder the guy who carelessly dropped your vase.

But meditation is internal behavior. Because you are not acting on your impulses in meditation, you don't need to edit them. On the contrary, you want to let every impulse move through you so that you can learn from each one and receive its gifts of energy and passion. This is by far the hardest thing for almost anyone to get. But don't worry, you have years to become accustomed to it.

Let's go over that again: you are not acting out thoughts; you are savoring them, releasing the energy tied up in them, freeing that energy for your life. This gives you total freedom to experience any thought. There is little most people ever experience that is not outdone on the nightly news or in the movies.

The relaxation and calmness of meditation are the foundation, and with that you want to welcome every taboo thought, every inappropriate impulse, so that you don't have to expend the energy to block it out. This is how you get defragmented.

If you want meditation to be restful and renewing, then let it be a time when you don't edit yourself. Let whatever hasn't had a chance to express itself come to the foreground and be cherished. Let meditation be Open House for all parts of yourself, whether they are tame or wild. If you do not let your passions play through you, you will get bored and want to quit meditation.

SELF-CRITICISM

If you find that your thoughts are self-critical, the secret is this: do nothing. Witness the thoughts. Listen and look. Breathe. At first you will be involved in the criticism, really believing it. At some point, though, you will remember that you are meditating and then simply return to the home base of wherever your chosen focus is. Do not try to block the thoughts in any way. If anything, welcome them. Whatever comes into the expansive space of meditation is gradually transformed.

Then, after meditation, go take good care of yourself. Love yourself up: take a walk or a bath, or luxuriate in some way. Talk to a good friend. Over time, you will learn to let negative thoughts just flow through you with no resistance. You will learn from them, get the information and pointers they sometimes bring, and be grateful for their input.

Tip: Each of the Obstacles is an Ally in disguise. You will have to learn this for yourself, and it will take time. The learning is a lifelong adventure. Thoughts are your brain at work, and it's good that your brain works. Each emotion is a relationship between something in you and something in the outer world, and it is good to be related to the world. Even moods represent inner callings that need attending to.

This Is Your Brain at Work

Your brain has maybe a trillion neurons, with seventy trillion synaptic connections among the neurons—there's an entire universe in there, like the stars in the sky. They all glow, hum, and commune with one another in the most delicate symphony conceivable.

Neurons in all the different parts of the brain are continually talking to one another, swapping data, telling one another stories. When we are resting, our brains do deep work, sorting everything out, healing connections, forming networks connecting everywhere with everywhere, reevaluating all priorities, noticing what has been missed. This goes on during the restfulness of deep sleep and dreaming, and it goes on in a similar fashion during the restfulness of meditation. The difference is that you are conscious during meditation, so you notice, and you have to learn to flow with it.

There is no need to try to get the neurons to stop communicating. Anyway, you couldn't do it; there is no mute button for the human brain. The hum of all that activity is the hum of life. Life is the symphony you are listening to.

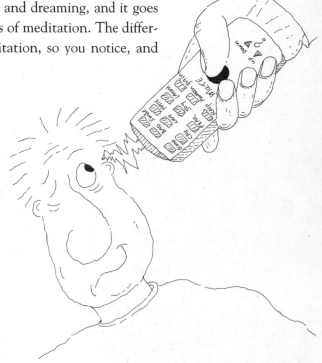

Remember this when you sit to meditate. During meditation, all the areas of the body and brain talk to one another even more than at other times, because you are resting and not doing anything else. Yet all this electricity, all this flowing of chemical messengers, is not an obstacle to meditation. This is your meditation. You can find the peace you crave amid this singing of neurons.

HOW MANY THOUGHTS DO YOU THINK IN AN HOUR?

Take a minute and notice how many thoughts you think. Then do the math and figure out how many per hour. Then calculate how many thoughts you think in the waking part of a day. What is it? Fifteen thousand? Twenty thousand? There is a tendency for thoughts to slow down or condense when you pay attention.

Depending on how busy you are, you may think a thousand or more thoughts an hour. If you like, you can count them, just as you do your pulse. It does not matter, though, whether the total is two hundred or fifteen hundred thoughts. The issue is, are you going to set your mind against the flow of thought or are you going to accept thought as part of meditation? Are you going to take the attitude that thoughts are not supposed to be there, or are you going to accept the flow of your thinking as part of the meditation?

If you do not accept thoughts wholeheartedly, then some part of you will have to set itself up as the Thought Police. Say you think extremely slowly—only a hundred thoughts an hour. But what if your Thought Police decides that is too many?

Say that after meditating for a few months, you think 20 percent fewer thoughts. Your mind is thinking more relevant, organized thoughts and has fewer random thoughts. This is likely, but the Thought Police will never be satisfied.

The brain is designed to think. If you find that you crave mental peace, embrace this craving and see where it leads. It leads to the ability to experience the quiet underneath thoughts. This occurs without repressing thought in any way. Essentially, what the meditator does is follow the flow of thoughts back to its source. Although thoughts do not stop, the experience of peace is very strong. It is as though a river of thought impulses is flowing through you, yet you can sit by the banks of this river and enjoy watching it flow.

Don't tell your brain to shut up. Instead, welcome all thoughts. This means welcoming even the thoughts you don't want, and the thought *Those other thoughts should not be there*, and the thought *Those thoughts should be controlled.*

You are not the Thought Police: "Attention all units. Racy thoughts entering limbic expressway at high speed." Meditation is not one set speed, such as slow. It is not slowing down. Your brain may speed up during meditation, or it may change speeds constantly. Your task as you go into meditation is to match your own natural motion and not get stuck in the role of traffic cop. You are not the police, telling everyone to slow down and striking fear in the hearts of speedsters and drivers of red sports cars. You are a musician in a jam session, a member of a band or symphony. Your task is to match rhythms, let them teach you their flow, join in, witness, learn how to pay attention to a vast and fast-moving enterprise.

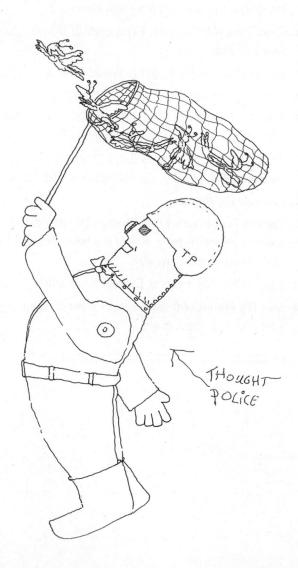

For People Who Must Have Rules: The Ten Commandments of Meditation

1. *Make Not Gods of Thy Gurus. If they have made gods of themselves, which is typical, then watch that you do not wind up a sacrifice on their altar.*

   Don't make meditation your religion. Let religion be religion and meditation the realm of pure experience.

2. *Thou Shalt Not Covet the Experience of Others. Be centered in your own self.*

3. *Do unto Your Inner Life as You Would Have It Do unto You.*

4. *Know Thy Preferences.*

5. *Beware of Those Who Would Enslave You in Their System. Let others waste money and time with the latest self-improvement fads.*

6. *Thou Shalt Not Delete Any Part of Thyself, No Matter How Troublesome. Work to bring the troublesome part into the fold.*

7. *Cultivate Thy Passions.*

8. *Validate Thy Individual Path Through This World. Rather than bow down to an image, be in awe of the infinite vastness of life. Salute that infinity in your own way.*

9. *Repress Not Thy Instincts. Express them within the legal limits.*

10. *Love Thy Breath. With each breath there is an ending of all that is past and a newness to life.*

◎ Welcoming Your Individuality

The Sense of Wonder

Wonder is very close to the essential spirit of meditation. If you simply think *Hmmm . . . I wonder what my approach to meditation is,* you will begin to get answers. I recommend spending one minute a day in wonder, perhaps before, during, or after reading a few pages of this book. Life and your own being will answer you over time. Give the question a couple of weeks, then let go of it and be alert to what your daily life shows you.

Whenever you ask a question of life, your whole nervous system seems to become oriented and alert for an answer. You can think of it as friendly angels guiding you, or you can think of it as your own hunting instincts being activated by your quest. The challenge of wonder is to tolerate uncertainty. If you do not relax into uncertainty, wonder may start to seem like insecurity.

I used to teach meditation techniques in a structured, step-by-step fashion, and I taught the same techniques to everyone, with only the tiniest modifications to accommodate people's individuality. One day in 1976 I changed the way I approached a session. Until then, I had been giving an instruction, waiting for the student to practice it a bit, then asking for a description of the experience. Based on that, I would give another instruction. But that day I started with a couple of questions instead of instructions. I said to a student, "In a while I'll give you some meditation instructions. But for now, let's just see what you normally, naturally experience when you pay attention to breathing." We sat there in the silence, breathing. A couple of minutes later I asked, "What interests you about breathing?" Then we sat for a few minutes with a sense of wonder and inquiry about breath.

After a while she took a deep breath and said, "Mmm . . . the flow-ingness of breath is such a pleasure. I can feel the air gliding in through my nose all the way to the depths of my belly, and then it turns and flows back out into the world." She was almost embarrassed at the inti-macy she was experiencing with breath, but she continued. One of the things she said was, "I feel that all of me is here, relaxed, poised, and ready for life. It is somehow an intense pleasure just to exist. I am at home in myself and at home in the world."

Over the next couple of minutes this young woman, who had no previous meditative experience, became completely absorbed in feel-ing the flow of breath. Perhaps because I waited patiently with no sense of hurry, she found the words to describe even the subtlest aspects of breath. With very little input from me, she became confi-dent in her ability to meditate and developed an intuitive grasp of the whole process and its rhythms. I never had to give her any direct instructions. I just kept asking questions and giving her a chance to experience for herself. Asking questions evoked her own ability to pay attention and devise her own techniques of meditation.

Mulling this over a few days later, I started laughing and the thought came to me, If people want to learn to meditate, who am I to get in their way?

Essentially, what I learned that day is that the body can teach us how to meditate if we give it a chance. Over the weeks and years that followed, I found out that most people can learn meditation in the same self-guided way. Everyone seems to have a way into meditation that is natural to him or her. Everywhere in the world I go, I meet self-taught meditators who have never studied with a teacher and who seem to be doing very well indeed.

As for the people who study with me on a regular basis, it seems that the essence of my work is to support them in being in wonder about their next step in life and in meditation. I encourage people to make up their program as they go along and check in with me as a reference, if they like. I have found, in thousands of interviews, that people have very good instincts for knowing what they need in meditation and how to get there. These self-guiding instincts come forward only when you are willing to engage your sense of wonder.

The Yoga of Needs

In learning to meditate from a book, you will look to your daily life as your arena. It is your individual needs, passions, and desires that have led you to want to meditate. And those same impulses will guide you. Ask yourself questions—what do I really want out of meditation? when in my day would I like to make time for it?—and take your time exploring the answers. What works for you may differ from what works for anyone else.

In the session described above, all I did was wonder about the unique way this person would go into meditation. That helped her feel safe to explore and to learn from her own experience of breath and silence. Even more important, I did not get in her way. She knew that I had answers if she really needed to ask about something, but because I did not fill the space with my knowledge, she activated her own self-guiding instincts. For me, doing sessions after that became an exercise in watching the human instinct for exploration. Over time I realized that many instincts come into play during meditation and while learning meditation: the homing instinct, self-preservation, healing instincts, and many more. Those instincts in you know your individual needs and how to satisfy them.

Your meditation technique will emerge from paying attention to your needs. You do this every time you allow your background sensations to come forward as you are getting into meditation. Your needs may present themselves as sensations of any kind anywhere in your body, as hankerings, lusts, images, desires, cravings, emotions, passions, and moods. Your practice is to feed each with attention, let it breathe, allow it to move through you.

A meditation technique is a relationship you establish between attentiveness and your needs. It is the link among all the elements of your life that want to come together so you can fulfill that need. This is yoga—yoga means linking together, and meditation is a type of "linking it all together" in the service of life.

In the years following 1976, I somehow accumulated a shelf of books on meditation that was more than forty feet long. It was just one long shelf running the length of the room, and it was jammed. There were books on meditation and spiritual practices from many traditions: Sufi, Yoga, Tibetan Buddhism, Chinese Taoism, Native American traditions, Zen, many different types of Western Occultism, Christian meditation, Jewish meditation, Egyptian mysteries, several schools of Sikh, the Hermetic tradition.

Listening to people tell me what they normally and naturally experience when they pay attention to breathing, I realized that people not only fall into meditation naturally, they spontaneously reinvent the classical meditation techniques in the books—even the most obscure ones. As people settle into their own style of meditation, just following their personal preferences, they find themselves paying attention in styles that were mapped out thousands of years ago—and there are many such styles. For one person, meditation may be like listening to a distant waterfall; for another, it may be like being outside under the stars, aware of the vastness and yet comforted by it. For others, the breath feels like lovemaking, massage, or feeding. Some people experience meditation as an awakening, as if all the unused parts of the self come alive and are then available to enjoy life. Many people, when they listen to the silence, hear singing sounds that shape themselves into mantras—the same mantras I would give those people if I had thought about it.

A problem for meditators is that when they are doing their native, most natural meditation, it doesn't feel like they are *doing* anything. Hundreds of times people have said to me, "That can't be my meditation technique! I feel like I am just sitting here being myself!" And yet one minute earlier that person was saying, "I feel perfectly at home in myself—rooted here on this spot and yet somehow aware of the universe. I can feel the sky above me. The universe seems friendly, somehow. I feel transparent, as if I am a galaxy—billions of tiny lights in a velvet emptiness."

When I had my library available, I would open one of the hundreds of books and find a technique that sounded just like what the person had said. It might be from a tradition he had never heard of, a Brahma sutra or a Sikh listening meditation. There is a different feeling tone to each tradition, as there is to different genres of music or different styles of cooking. Within that feeling tone are innumerable recipes. Your inner feeling tone for meditation may be something that has lived on Earth at some time and been recorded, or it may not have been recorded. It may not even have been felt before. The range is huge: hundreds of major ways.

As you become familiar with meditation, engage more and more with your individual taste. Celebrate it. Seek out music, theater, novels, movies, poetry, and people that affirm your own experience of life and meditation.

Surprise

Being willing to be surprised is another essential meditation attitude. Willingness to be surprised is more than not having expectations. It is a willingness to be shocked, startled, delighted, appalled, amazed, grieved, and grateful at what you feel and see and hear inside yourself. It is a trust you extend to your inner life that leads you to release control. In meditation you are meeting the universe in a new way. You will get relaxation no matter what, and you will get a kind of serenity. You can take that for granted. But you may as well be willing to be electrified as well. It is always a challenge to accept your full electricity in meditation, because the tone of it changes in small ways from day to day, and in major ways over a period of months.

Be Willing to Be Surprised

Feeling the Movement of Your Life

Meditation is about feeling the urges, impulses, and impetus of your life. It is about centering yourself in life's flow, living in the calm inner center, coming back to center again and again, endlessly. It is not just

> *Tip: Remember—meditation is not about slowing down. Meditation gives you the ability to speed up as well as to slow down. You will also know your body's rhythm more intimately. You will be better able to move at your own pace. Everyone's pace is different. Often in meditation, the brain seems to speed up, thoughts race around for a while, then suddenly there's stillness. It's unpredictable.*

focusing; it is returning to the focus, then losing it and returning, again and again.

Life is energy and substance in motion, an exquisite dance. Our daily life is part of the vast dance of Life on Earth and the Earth Orbiting the Sun. Meditation is about silently feeling your connection to all this. The silence and peace are not a lack of movement; they are balancing in the midst of movement. Faster vibrations can even feel more peaceful.

All this is voluntary. It has to be. To stay in meditation is to invite life to flow through you more intensely. It is to invite life to change, remodel, update you.

Honoring the Inner Rebel

You never know where the spiritual part of you is hidden. Because this is meditation, and not the army, your impulse to rebel against discipline is as important as your desire to change yourself for the better. You may have noticed in the past that when you try to get yourself to do a self-help program, you wind up tyrannizing yourself. Then you rebel against the tyranny. The rebel becomes a saboteur of your program because you left her out. The way through this is to embrace the rebel right from the start.

Welcoming the rebel may mean listening to the feeling *I don't want to meditate today* and finding out what it wants. To honor such a feeling means to take it so seriously that you would be willing not to meditate but to watch TV instead, or watch the sunset. But you are also willing to enter the feeling, explore it, let it teach you. Welcome the rebellion, then listen to it. The rebel is there to make sure you do not become enslaved in an external system that takes away your inner authority, restricts your inner freedom, or oppresses you in any way.

Meditating the rebel's way may seem strange. Once I was working with a schoolteacher, and she was getting restless just a few minutes into her first session. When I asked, "What are your impulses?" she said, "I just want to be outside." We went outside, and since we were on a mountain in northern New Mexico, we could see vast horizons. She breathed a sigh of relief. It turned out that she prefers to be outside as much as possible, even in winter. She dresses warmly, sits in the snow, and has a great time meditating. The rebel in her is her spiritual part. Another woman's rebel might insist that she sit cozily in bed to meditate on certain days.

The rebel in you is probably smarter, healthier, and more useful than your impulse to practice meditation. Many people, when they imagine meditating, conceive of it as some sort of inner prison. Your inner rebel will immediately alert you if you start making up Odious Rules such as "You can't think, you can't feel, you can't scratch if you itch." The rebel will have none of this. The way in which you rebel is your individuality.

So honor your inner rebel. As you do the meditations, be alert for the voice of skepticism in you, the voice that says, *Hey, wait a minute, this is bull!* The rebel looks out for your individuality. Invite it in, no matter how much trouble it seems.

As you read about and explore meditation, notice anything you hate or don't want to do. Always take your own side. Be willing to hunt for your own particular way.

Embracing All Parts of the Self

The greatest danger for meditators is deleting parts of the self. The parts of yourself that you snub and do not invite to the party cannot give you their gifts. When you delete parts of the self, you limit your vitality and your range of expression. In the long run, this will mean that you either go through life as an overly peaceful meditator or quit meditating because you have made meditation a kind of prison.

Think of meditation as a party you are giving for every aspect of your humanity, every aspect of the soul. Invite even the street people, the witchy bitch, the cranky skeptic, though they seem incongruous.

Maybe they stink and don't know how to use the silverware, but feed them. When any quality is integrated, when it gets to rub shoulders with all the other parts of the self, it changes and is socialized. Each has a gift to give you.

What part of yourself have you lost? It could be a feeling tone from your schooldays—perhaps you were athletic or you sang in the shower a lot. It could be the movie lover in you or the letter writer. The purpose of life is to get survival taken care of so that we can get on with being as individualistic as possible. Many men lose the lover in them when they hunker down to work long hours. In the process of gearing up to be successful, people often find that they have lost the person inside who was capable of enjoying the success. If you continue meditating, you can be sure that the lost parts of you will come knocking at the door to be let in. They may appear as moods, images, memories, or sensations in your body. Welcome them, even though you most likely will not know what they are at first.

In fairy tales, it is the unpleasant aunt, the one not invited to the wedding, who shifts into a malevolent witch and curses the marriage.

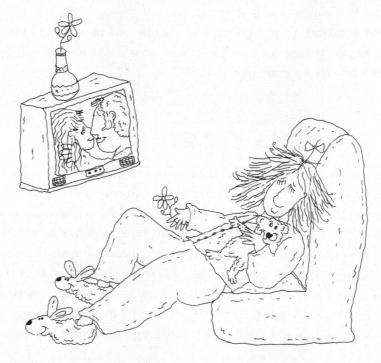

When people go into meditation with a spiritual approach, you can almost hear the ripping sound as they split off parts of themselves to fit their picture of what a proper meditator is. It is a kind of Peter Pan syndrome, in which the Shadow is split off and then becomes Other.

In meditation, you have a few months to get used to the range of your inner experience and train yourself to accept it all—or not. The habits you develop will tend to be permanent. This is what I see in my friends and in the people who come to me for coaching. The attitude with which they went into meditation has become cast in concrete. At some point, a necessary crisis was missed.

In everyday life, we have to edit our responses to match what is appropriate in the environment. This is healthy. Each of us has a set of emotions that we allow and a set that we disallow—this is called a personality. When you begin meditation you have a fresh start on life, on how you slice up the pie of your inner qualities. If you just carry over your outer-world adaptation to the inner world, you miss much of the opportunity meditation offers. You do the equivalent of taking your elementary school personality over into high school.

Anger, greed, sexuality, revenge, ambition, wild passionate adoration of anything, the desire to be drunk or Dionysian, fear, laziness—which of these do you have trouble with? Which of these do you think are not a proper part of meditation?

Whatever you leave out cannot be integrated. It sounds obvious when put that way. Remember, though, that in meditation all your thoughts and feelings are whizzing through your body and nerves at high speed, and it will take you quite a while to learn what they are. The acceptance of all parts of yourself has to translate to the level of reflex. This comes only from gradually developing trust—trust of the space of meditation, trust of your body, trust of what the nervous system is, trust of what your brain is, trust in life itself.

Your task is to take the embracing attitude from the level of theory to the level of your bodily responses. During meditation, things happen too fast for theory. You operate out of reflex. That is why I say meditation is more a physical sport than a mental game. Or you could say it is more like a relationship with all your parts. If a child playing in the backyard turns from her little world and comes running to you to share her excitement about a caterpillar she has been watching, you have less than a second to decide to accept her embrace even though she is muddy and you are wearing nice clothes. If you stop to think, *Hmm . . . okay, this is my niece, and she is in an explosion of enthusiasm for life and discovery that I cannot ever hope to return to. Every moment of her three-year-old life is a major moment. Do I let her get my clothes dirty or do I try to hold her at arm's length?* she will see your hesitation or disgust or preoccupation, and that is what she will get. You will miss the magic of the moment. Or you could embrace her with open arms, share in her joy, and she would run back to her play fulfilled. What moves you toward this kind of emotional suppleness with yourself and others? Is it music, theater, movies, friends, conversations? Find out and cultivate it. Go on in and make friends. Get muddy.

Sex, Drugs, and Rock 'n' Roll

All of us have at least one secret desire that we consider sinful according to some scheme of things. Something that feels like a vice. You may have had experiences being wild at concerts or drinking and dancing all night. You may recall times when you felt really good being bad.

Every vice has a secret to teach us. The secret is in the desire for a certain quality of experience: intensity, freedom, wildness, vivid colors, aliveness, total joy, free-flowing sexuality, innocence, a heightening of the senses, universal love, lack of inhibition. These are all good qualities. There is much to be said for each. As a matter of fact, they are much too important to be left to chance, or to imported illegal substances, or to complicated arrangements of people. Using substances to experience these qualities can physically destroy you. Face up to it, drugs are obsolete.

Meditation is for passions and cravings so deep they can't be fulfilled by ordinary experience. All of us have desires that can't be fulfilled—we want to live forever, be perfectly thin or muscular, have unlimited money, be on vacation eternally, have all the love in the world. In meditation you ride these cravings and they take you into some level of life where the joy of movement is itself enough delight; where it is better to be in movement, playing with life, at peace inside yourself, than it is to have arrived at any goal.

Even the ancient word *meditarai*, from which our word *meditation* is derived, speaks of this connection of mindfulness, rhythm, and the harmony that heals. All this means that meditation is an interior Sex, Drugs, and Rock 'n' Roll. The sex is the passionate current of desire. It's subtle, but sexy. Relaxation is very sexy, and most people get turned on when they are deeply relaxed. The drugs part is the body's own internal pharmacy as it heals itself. Dozens of scientific studies have shown dramatic drops in the stress chemicals and increases in the natural opiates during meditation. The rock 'n' roll is the inner music, the pulsation of the heartbeat and breath. The harmony can be a measure of music, a measured sound such as a mantra, or exactly the right song played at the right moment to satisfy the soul. The meditation traditions of the world have explored ways of paying attention to flow, pulsation, and inner songs so that you never tire of them but actually get more and more interested.

Don't Judge Yourself

Meditation is taking the same circuits you use when you are having a good time and then underwhelming yourself. We should be bored, but we aren't. In this delicious underloading of the senses, something magical happens. When you do this, when you let yourself be shaped by these moments, your whole body and heart and mind realign with life. Believe it or not, this is what the sacred traditions have been saying for thousands of years.

The ecstatic longing to be transported is the same whether we are at a rock concert or an opera, watching our favorite television show or in a totally silent meditation room. The main difference is that in meditation you follow the impulses of pleasure beyond themselves into the silence, and you rest there. In meditation you learn to respond more and more to less and less, so that the quieter the music is, the more intensely you feel it. In meditation even the simple action of breathing or listening to the rhythm of the vowel sounds becomes intensely pleasurable.

Meditation is not taking something away or denying ourselves something. Meditation is adding something: the willingness to follow the music into the silence; to follow the beat into the space between beats; to follow the rhythm of breath into the great interior dance.

Exercises for Uncovering Your Personal Style

THE RHYTHM OF EVERYDAY LIFE

Let's take a minute to recognize some elements of your personal style. Just take a conscious break in the midst of all this reading and ask yourself some pertinent questions. We've been talking about the importance of asking and the magic of the answers just percolating up. So now, consider the rhythm of your everyday life and the pace at which you like to move.

- Do you like to move fast, have the feeling that lots of things are happening simultaneously?

- Do you prefer a slow, orderly pace to life?

- What rhythms turn you on? Slow and sultry? Dynamic and energetic? Lyrical and soulful?

- Is your personal aesthetic minimalist, simple, spare? Extravagant, colorful, outrageous? Somewhere in between?

Once you ask, you'll know. Now the best advice I can ever give you is to learn to meditate without cramping your own style. It may seem odd to meditate for only half a minute and then stop to make sure you are not making a chore of it or putting pressure on yourself in some way. But by doing so, you will be developing ease, rhythm, and a sense of your individual style. Then you can do longer and longer meditations and feel comfortable. Any one meditation of ten or twenty minutes is composed of many minute to minute-and-a-half cycles. A lot happens in a minute.

To keep it simple, I suggest that you approach meditation with an appreciation of movement. Attention moves, whether you want it to or not, so by accepting this in advance you will not be at war with yourself.

- If you like to move fast, the best way for you to approach meditation is by doing quickies: quick in and out; doing each meditation for a short time, so it seems like a brief but satisfying pit stop in the racecourse of your life.

- If you like to have a leisurely pace whenever possible, set aside a chunk of time, and give lots of attention to the getting-in and getting-out phases.

- If you know you love rhythm, if you love the way your body feels in the presence of drums or a band with a great beat, play music and dance to it before you meditate. You don't have to do this every time, but when you do, you'll find that the delicious, erotic energy of the rhythm permeates your meditation and touches deep into your core.

- If you crave simplicity or silence, give it to yourself. Seek out times and places of quiet, so your nerves can thrive on the sanctuary that silence gives.

- If you find yourself craving rich colors and complex imagery, experiment with meditating in a Catholic church or an art museum.

YOUR RULING PASSIONS

You do not have to give up any passions to meditate; on the contrary, you celebrate them even more, following the trail they have made in your nerves and body. The peacefulness and tolerance of meditation are complemented by the richness of experience represented in wild vices.

What is this desire we all share, to move with abandonment, to numb out some pain, to be intensely stimulated? Whatever the vice, there is a legitimate calling behind it. Use meditation to explore that calling.

Consider the following questions. Ask them silently to yourself and then listen for your answers. Call up your memory. You may even be moved to speak them out loud. Come on—you won't be arrested.

- What is my favorite vice?
- What is a vice I loved but had to give up?
- What is the best I have ever felt while doing some wild and sinful activity?

Now feel the excitement, the relaxation, the expanded awareness, the sexual intensity flowing through your nervous system. Allow yourself to have the fullness of that without getting into trouble, just sitting there on your sofa or in your meditation chair.

In case you've blanked out some possible vices, here's a quick list for easy reference!

- Smoking cigarettes.
- Smoking pot.
- Drinking a lot at parties and dancing all night.
- Doing cocaine or other drugs.
- Overeating.
- Having lots of sex or naughty sex.

These are Dionysian forms of worship, celebrations of the passions. When you go inside and cherish the experience of wildness, it becomes an Apollonian meditation—contained and outwardly respectable, because nobody can see what you're thinking. You don't have to stop feeling wild inside just because you aren't acting out anymore.

◎ Meditation in Your Daily Life

How Do I Let Meditation Be Easy?

Ease is defined as "rest, quiet, and repose." Ease is "freedom from work." Ease is also informality and release from constraint. This is a pretty good description of meditation! Meditation is a time when you are not pressuring yourself to perform. You are resting very deeply and relaxing, yet you are paying attention in an easy manner.

Ease is actually a requirement for both learning and practicing meditation. That's because when you try to pay attention, only a tiny part of your being is involved in the "trying." Meditation involves paying attention with your entire being.

If you catch yourself "working at it," stop instantly. Take a breath, shake yourself out, stretch, open your eyes, do anything to interrupt the pattern. Working at meditation is the one big boo-boo.

Meditation is a built-in ability. All human beings have it innately. The techniques are ways of giving the body permission to enter meditation, which it wants to do anyway. When you find the times and ways that your body naturally wants to meditate, then meditation really does feel easy.

When you think about meditation, put it in the same category of things you do just because you feel like it, whether it is dancing, making love, fishing, talking on the phone to your friends, or going to a movie. Do you tend to put meditation above your head, as if it were spiritual? Spirituality is just one of the many tones of meditation, and it is not the most important one by any means.

When do you have the greatest sense of ease in life? What are you doing when you feel easy? Do you have special activities or times in the week for cultivating ease?

Another way to let meditation be easy is to choose techniques and senses you are interested in. There are hundreds of things to meditate on. Entire worlds of meditation techniques have been developed for fighting, making love, eating, hunting, painting, listening to music, healing painful memories, and exploring the subtle planes of existence. Any one person may not have time to explore fully all the meditation practices for each instinct, but you will have many of these interests going on in your life at any one time. And your meditation, no matter what technique you use, will have elements of fighting, sex, nourishment, hunting, and art. You will find that you pay attention quite easily to what you are interested in. As you explore meditation, your challenge will be to let your practice be shaped by your inner needs as they emerge.

Think of any good book or movie or play or opera you have ever loved. There is actually a meditation technique about that type of drama. The only difference is that in meditation the drama is approached from the inside. The yogis and meditation traditions have been interested in what parts of the body, what chakras or energies are employed by or represented by each character. How do the energy centers in the body work together or fight one another in the course of such a conflict?

Let's say you sit to meditate at the end of the day after work. Your first experience may be total relief: *Ah, how blessed just to sit here.* But after a few minutes of relaxation, you may find that your brain is generating thoughts about the power dynamics at work. Is my job threatened? Will I have to move to the new office building across town? As these thoughts flow through your awareness, your body is practicing staying relaxed, and sometimes failing to do so. Your body and brain will bring up worrisome situations again and again until you can stay relaxed all the way through. Relaxed here means that you are not running scared; you have the presence of mind to consider all your options, and you do not think that your life is threatened when it is only your status in this temporary tribe.

This process can be painful. Each time you think of your boss, you may feel your solar plexus jump. Dare I ask for a raise? In reality, however, this is your own personal movie you are watching. It is your favorite novel, the one in which you are the protagonist. Every drama you have ever seen or read is there to help you understand and act within the plot structure of your life. Meditation is the time when you, as hero or heroine of your own drama, in the midst of your daily life, take a moment to charge your batteries and emerge renewed. Your thought process, the whole struggle to face your challenges with your senses and heart open, is really the most interesting thing around. You will learn this from your own daily meditation practice. It really is quite interesting to sit there and breathe and watch the plot of your day unfold before your mind's eye. Then in twenty minutes or so you get up and you are a little freer, as if you have just come back from vacation.

Remember: One way to let meditation be easy and keep it simple is to make it about your needs, about helping you to fulfill your immediate needs, such as the need for rest, the need to be able to focus well at work, the need to be able to relax while under pressure, the need to communicate clearly. This keeps the whole enterprise of meditation honest, because you will be able to tell each day how you are doing, how well your meditation is working. No Hindu metaphysics or Tibetan mysteries are involved.

Another way to allow meditation to be easy is to not be artificial with yourself in any way. Ease is defined as informality, freedom from constraint, freedom from labor, naturalness. In sailing there is a term, *ease off,* that means to back off from running too close to the wind. If you want meditation to be restful, a solace for your soul, and a place of renewal, learn to be easy with yourself in meditation. Being easy with yourself and easing off is a kind of a physical skill that you can practice. You can do it with each breath. While meditating, you will probably catch yourself occasionally trying too hard and need to ease off.

> **Tip:** If you find yourself in a long series of thoughts, you sometimes have the option to pay attention to the sensations underlying the thoughts. If you scan your body, you may find that you have sensations in your throat, heart, or belly that correspond to the emotional dramas your brain is sorting through. Let your attention be called there, and breathe with the sensations.

GUIDELINES FOR YOUR PERSONAL MEDITATION

Refer to this list of guidelines if you feel lost, confused, over-whelmed, worried, obsessed, or simply need to get a grip.

Remember . . .

- Follow your own rhythms.
- Welcome all your thoughts and feelings, especially uncomfortable ones.
- Greet your inner rebel, the part of you that may say, *I don't want to meditate*.
- Honor your preferences. Let your meditation be like your natural self, your natural cravings, your own set of needs.
- Never force anything in meditation. Learn what effortlessness is. There is plenty of room for effort in the outer world.
- Whenever you begin a meditation, just sit there for a couple of minutes and let your nerves settle in.
- Welcome all the experiences you will ever have and those you have never even dreamed of.
- Honor your discomfort. Much of your meditation time will be spent massaging the sore areas of your life, reviewing mistakes, healing inner wounds, accessing relaxation, and then mentally rehearsing action.
- Take refuge in meditation but do not use it to numb yourself.
- Do not tell your mind to shut up. Inner noise is not noise. Thoughts come and go.
- Increase your tolerance for creative tension, for all that is unsolved. Use meditation to give you the courage to face your unsolved issues.
- Learn to tolerate the unstressing process—the painful process of your body letting go of tension.
- Make meditation a generous space, one that includes all of who you might ever be. Cry, laugh, dissolve, let go, rage, worry, go insane, be wild, want to kill your enemies, want to die, want to be saved.

- Meditation should feel like a luxurious indulgence, at least much of the time.

- If your mind wanders, don't hit it. A wandering mind is not a problem, but any effort or strain is.

- You will never experience the same thing twice. Therefore, don't expect anything in particular to happen.

- Break the rules. Make up your own rules. Customize your meditation.

- Sleep is not a problem. If you get sleepy, lie down.

- Speed is not a problem. You do not have to slow down.

- Judge by how you feel an hour or two after meditation. Notice how well you do in your essential life tasks, in work, in relationship, in nature, in sleep.

Don't Furrow Your Brow

When people talk socially, you can see them gesturing, moving their eyes as they speak. If you ask a friend a question, he may look up and to the side or down and to the side. It's as if people are inside their minds, inside their own amphitheater of thinking. This is the normal unconstrained mode, in which we have plenty of room. In general, most people scowl only when they are angry, and then only briefly.

When "meditating," though, people often abandon their natural mode and try to constrict or "concentrate" their minds. You can tell because they furrow their brows. You might have a friend peek in on you when you are meditating sometime and let you know if you are furrowing your brow. If you are, do brief mini-meditations and take walks or naps instead of meditating. Do not let this habit set in.

Tip: Watch basketball or another sport in which the players are running around keeping track of many fast-moving bodies. Look at the expression on the players' faces—they are almost blank with total concentration.

Customizing Your Meditation

How do I choose what my meditation is going to be this day, this week, this month?

If these were the old days, you might go to a guru and he would tell you. You would not need to have any self-knowledge. Or the priest would tell you, "Ten Hail Marys, ten Our Fathers."

You have instincts to know what you want and need. Think of the way you select music to listen to when you are alone, or the way you know you need water when you feel the sensation called thirst. Whenever you pay attention to your body, you will get guidance.

Look over the list below. Each type of meditator on the list is an example of some craving, some ruling passion or instinct. What are yours?

Twenty Types of Meditators

REBEL: "To hell with the world, this is my time."

MUSICIAN: "I am going to listen to the silence and music of my being."

SENSUALIST: "Ahhhhh . . . this is like a massage."

CAT: "Zzzzzzz and purrrrr."

GOURMET: "Ah, what delicious air; this is better than chocolate."

SEEKER: "I am searching for the lost parts of my true self."

SURFER: "This is a blast, surfing the waves of my mind."

LOVER: "I am going to go into my heart and feel all the longing and ecstasy there."

BOSS: "I am going to take charge around here. Clean up that mind! Organize those dreams!"

CRITICAL BYSTANDER: "What a mess this mind is! Whose thoughts are these anyway? What is that thought doing there?"

GARDENER: "This is like watering the plants and pulling weeds. Maybe I'll put this thought here on the compost heap."

EXHAUSTED LABORER: "It is pure relief just to sit still for a few minutes."

DANCER: "Meditation is movement, inner worlds of movement."

DREAMER: "I am lying back, looking at the clouds moving across the vast sky of my mind."

MYSTIC: "I am going to penetrate the mysteries of life."

HEALER: "I have compassion for the whole world and all the wounded people walking around in it."

WANDERER: "Take me into new realms of experience, take me traveling."

ARTIST: "I meditate for the pure joy of the colors, shapes, and textures revealed to me."

SLAVE: "I am a speck in God's creation."

SCIENTIST: "I want to know how things work, and I am going to perform meditation as an experiment to gather data."

Notice what your approach is—or approaches. You may relate to two, three, or even more. Feel free to expand the list in any way, and mail me your additions.

You may have one of these as your primary ego and one as your alter ego. Alter egos are like subpersonalities, each with its own needs, preferences, and style of meditating. Just ask them—they'll tell you what they want!

They are all doorways into meditation.

JOHN DISCOVERS HIS NATURAL STYLE

The key to developing a meditation that fits your life is to move with your own natural tone, speed, and rhythm of attention. Follow the same natural movement of attention you engage in when you are having a good time doing something you love. Don't violate the integrity of your style, and do not repress your impulses, no matter how wild. Most of us have tendencies to repress our wild impulses; doing so is useful in the outer world but stultifying in meditation.

Meditation is different from the waking state. It is a separate state in which you don't act on impulses but merely witness them as they move through you. If you don't let them arise, however, there is nothing to witness but your repression, and then meditation goes stale. If you find yourself struggling in meditation, inquire into the fine details of what you are experiencing. Go in there and look closely at what is there and what you think you are supposed to do, and you will find the solution. Let's look at an example.

John had a strong urge to meditate and felt that he needed some instruction. When he came by for a meditation session, I noticed that within seconds of closing his eyes, he would start to frown slightly. He was very strong, with tremendous vitality, so I was curious to know what had him scowling. I asked him to close his eyes. A few seconds later, I said, "What are you experiencing? What does it feel like?"

It took several minutes, then he said, "I am in a vast open space and thoughts are flying everywhere," and he frowned again.

Then I asked, "How many different directions are the thoughts moving in?"

He seemed surprised as he looked inside himself to track the thoughts. "All directions, left to right, up to down, right to left . . ." I could see his eyes moving behind his eyelids.

I could tell from his complexion that John spent a good deal of time outdoors, so I asked, "Have you ever stood outdoors and watched a storm blowing in from the ocean and simply enjoyed the movement of the clouds? And the continual change in the light . . . [speaking slowly] the cooling of the air, the first drops . . ."

This turned out to be a good guess on my part, because he started smiling and said, "Yes, I have. Many times. I love rain and wind and clouds. I love to watch weather coming in over the sea."

So I said, "Treat your inner experience just as you would the weather. When you want to absorb the vitality of it, go ahead and stand in it and enjoy every movement."

What I implied by my questions and suggestion was that John could enjoy his inner experience just as much as he enjoyed the weather. This was the first step: that he just accept with pleasure something vast, unpredictable, and moving. He had been thinking of meditation as "going inside" and therefore had decided that he needed to constrict his attention somehow. I also indirectly suggested that his inner world could be as vast and unconstrained as the outer world he loves. He had been trying to condense his attention and "fix" it into a small internal space. Maybe he felt he had to squeeze his essence to fit it inside his skull. His natural sense of himself was already expanded, and he was trying to shrink it.

My metaphor also implied that going in and facing the inner weather was like standing outside and welcoming the weather blowing in. I knew from his facial expression that he did not cower from the rain but rejoiced in it. I gave him permission to take his physical joy and "no problem" attitude in dealing with the elements and map them over to his inner world. And I indicated that he could take shelter from his inner experience whenever he wanted. This gave him control over how much he wanted to face. I used these metaphors to break up his old habit of attention and his model of what meditation was, since that model was violating his natural style.

You can see from this example how people dumb themselves down in the name of meditation. John had spontaneously meditated many times, particularly when camping out. He loved to stay awake as much of the night as possible, just watching the stars and savoring the vastness of space. He was already an advanced "spontaneous meditator." But now he wanted to be able to access that kind of feeling in town or wherever he was. The problem was in his mental model of meditation, which cramped his style. His habit of frowning and trying to corral his attention could have started in kindergarten, or the first time he had to sit in a tiny chair and read a children's book when he would rather have been outside running around.

One of the instructions I gave John was "Breathe with the vastness. Enjoy your breathing as a gift from the world's oceans, the forests, and the sun." This immediately made breathing ecstatic to him. Meditation became a tremendous pleasure, and he could take moments here and there throughout the day to breathe, in addition to doing more formal meditations. John already knew vastness—he just needed to accept it.

John then took the lesson a step farther, into something I had not even thought about. It turned out that he sometimes got really mad when people violated his boundaries or did something unethical. His anger would flash wildly. Since he now had the sense of his inner space as vast, the anger could be experienced as lightning. He learned to enjoy the power of the lightning and to enjoy having a choice about whether to express it. But he no longer felt he needed to repress it: it wasn't an either/or choice of flying off the handle or stuffing it. He could feel powerful and grounded when angry, then choose how to act.

If John had kept meditating with his scowl, he probably would have had a rough go at it, then quit. And it would have been better to quit than to continue to cramp his own style of paying attention. He could have developed headaches, and he certainly would have lost vitality. Instead of carrying over his richness of experience, he was impoverishing himself by the way he was attempting to pay attention.

Meditation is subtle internal behavior, and very few people ever get adequate coaching. It takes hours of careful instruction to undo the bad habits most people fall into, whether they learn meditation in a yoga class, from a book, in a workshop, or somewhere else. You can do for yourself what I do with the people who come to me, and save yourself a lot of trouble. Just go step-by-step, and breathe as you read the book. Have a good time and don't force anything. Meditate less than you want to for weeks or months, so that you always look forward to the next time. It is much better to take an all-embracing attitude toward your inner experience in the first place. I have so many friends who have been meditating for decades and have never undone the bad habits with which they started. You do not need to follow such a path. This book contains all the clues you need, and you will get them one at a time, little by little, as you make meditation your own.

The Eight Acceptances

1. *Accept the Rhythm of Your Experience.*
2. *Accept the Blues.*
3. *Accept the Motion of Emotion, Desire, and Passion.*
4. *Accept All Parts of the Self.*
5. *Accept the Wisdom of the Instincts.*
6. *Accept the Play of Universality and Individuality.*
7. *Accept Surprise and Uncertainty.*
8. *Accept Your Boundaries and Grow Beyond Them.*

Daily Life Meditations

Here are some recipes for including meditation in the cycle of your day. Mix and match as you like. Pick one, two, or three from among the choices. You will invent your own routines. The exciting thing to discover is how much you can change your bodily state for the better in a brief period of time.

To Start the Day

Be Cozy

Wake Up and Smell the Coffee

Hot-Cold Shower

Opening Ritual

Heart Meditation

Explore the Vowels

Arrive Early

To Refresh Yourself During the Day

Take a Breather

Slump Exercise

What Do You Really Love

Inhale and Hold

Salute the Senses (especially Hearing and Sight)

To Settle Down

(When stress is getting to you or you feel overwhelmed)

Do Nothing

Tense to Relax

Match Rhythms with Yourself

Fast Breath

Slow Exhale

Ah-Hum

Give In to Gravity

Perfect Safety Exercise
Salute the Sense of Touch

To Get Charged Up

Fast Breath
Breathe Power
Pause at a Threshold
Chant the Vowel Sounds
Salute the Sense of Balance
Give In to Gravity
What's Up

To Unwind

(At the end of the day, after work)

Stretch
Do Nothing
Give In to Gravity
Welcome a Breath
Stillness in Motion
Let Your Brain Go Limp
Ra-Ma

To Prepare for a Social Evening

Hot-Cold Shower
Take a Conscious Nap
All Senses Meditation (especially Smell, Taste, and Touch)
Heart Meditation
Breathe Power

To End the Day

Review the Day

Before-Sleep Meditation
Be Cozy
Slow Exhale

IF YOU ARE AWAKE AT NIGHT

Sometimes when we've had a lot going on during the day, our nervous system gets wired and sleep eludes us. Or we wake up in the middle of the night, begin worrying about not getting enough zzz's, and drive ourselves crazy trying to fall asleep again.

Here are some suggestions for relaxing before bed:

- Take a hot bath.
- Don't eat a lot late at night.
- Turn off the TV half an hour before bedtime. In general, watch only comedy shows in the evening. Don't load your brain with junk information before going to sleep.
- Give yourself some transition time before going to sleep. Do the Review of the Day meditation and lay your day to rest. Get in your pj's (if you wear them) and hang out on the bed for a while. When you do slip under the covers, let yourself feel their comfort and safety welcoming you. Do a Before-Sleep or Be Cozy meditation.

If you still find yourself waking up at 3:00 A.M., do not struggle. I recommend two complementary attitudes: get interested in your sensory impressions, and, strangely enough, get interested in your thoughts. The middle of the night is a natural meditation time, a time when life catches up with us, trying to get our attention in some way. I often have my most creative insights in the middle of the night.

So there you are, wide awake. What do your senses tell you? What pleasure can you be aware of? Feel the soft texture of your pillow, the coziness of your sheets and blankets. There's the feeling of your body weight being supported by the bed. You can just let yourself drop into gravity, like falling into an embrace from the Earth. In the quiet of the

night, most of life's creatures are regenerating; there in a velvet darkness, rich and soothing. In your body there is the ongoing ebb and
flow of the breath, like the gentle swell of ocean waves, rising, falling,
rising, falling . . .

Maybe you feel your nerves buzzing, which you associate with anxiety. What if you recognize that buzz as life force moving through you
with electricity, and let yourself ride the pathways of current? Is there
something pleasurable in that feeling? The idea here is to accept what
you can of your experience, so that you don't compound your sleepless-
ness by beating yourself up.

One meditator writes, "I often spend hours at night in this limbo
land of attention, especially when I'm hot on the trail of some creative
project. So I let my body relax as much as possible while my mind does
its thing. That way, I am still getting physical rest even as my thoughts
are working something out. I have come to savor these middle-of-the-
night meditations."

Beauty. Safety. Surrender. Welcome all thoughts. Bless your dreams
in advance. Leap into the unknown.

What the Word Meditation Really Means

Meditation comes from a family of words having to do with healing,
balance, music, rhythm, harmony, measure, and paying attention. The
Latin word *meditarai* means to attend, to be present, to look after, heal,
cure. This mosaic of meaning points to meditation as the process of
paying attention to the underlying harmony of life so that balance is
restored. Even if you think etymology is boring, check out the richness
of meanings in the word *meditation*.

The *med* of meditation is an ancient Indo-European root word
meaning "to take appropriate measures." Indo-European is the proto-
language from over seven thousand years ago that gave rise to Sanskrit, Indic, Iranian, Slavic, Albanian, Anatolian, Greek, Latin, Ger-
man, and eventually English. Many of the words we use every day
derive from Indo-European roots.

A number of our commonly used words are based on the root *med:*

model, meter, medicine, remedy, meditate, modest, modern, accommodate, must, and empty (*American Heritage Dictionary of the English Language*, 1992, Houghton Mifflin Company).

Meter is the beat or rhythm, and *medicine* is the balance. Thus meditation is the harmony that heals, the music that heals you and restores balance.

Being *modest* involves knowing exactly who you are, being neither inflated nor deflated.

Model refers to the template you are working from to build your life.

Modern means "just now," current, what is happening.

Modify is to refine the design, make it better.

Accommodate is what we must learn to do constantly, accommodate ourselves and the world.

Empty is the way space itself feels; emptiness is the arena for life. Things aren't crowded together—there is enough emptiness or space in our houses, our heads, between us and the movie screen.

Just looking in the dictionary, you can see the rich spectrum of what *meditation* means and how the word is related to things you already know.

Each of these meanings will become vitally important to you if you continue exploring meditation. In one twenty-minute meditation you may find yourself feeling harmonious, then feeling alternately depressed and exhilarated for a few minutes, then balancing out in a steady knowing of who you are. A minute later you are electrified by a vivid awareness of the current of your life and how exciting that is. The excitement may then turn to fear as you wonder if you are up to some task ahead of you. Then your body works through the fear and massages calmness into it. Your mind turns to focus on where you are in your life and how time is passing. You may alternate between feeling full and empty, full of memories and experiences or empty and hungry. In fact, this is a pretty typical set of qualities experienced by almost any meditator in any meditation. Meditation is accommodating yourself, being accommodating. It's being hospitable to your soul, all of it, every quality. I was very surprised to find all this wisdom about meditation technique just sitting there in the etymology section of a dictionary.

The Meditation Top Forty

Here are a few dozen meditation techniques from the Bhairava Tantra, the ancient Sanskrit meditation text I mentioned at the beginning of this book. Each of these techniques can be done for a few seconds at a time or for hours. Read a few now, or as many as you want, then return later. For many years I could not bear to read more than one or two at a sitting. Go at your own pace.

Notice the ones you are drawn to and the ones that remind you of awakenings you have already had.

1. Attend to life as flow. Nothing is fixed, everything flows.

2. Breath is continuous pulsation. Be at home in the eternal rhythm.

3. Breath moves through you, in and out, twenty-two thousand times a day. Set aside some time to consciously enjoy the beauty of that flowing. Give yourself a chance to fall in love with breath.

4. Breathing is something we do in cooperation with the whole world. It is a flowing exchange of substance with the ocean of air that surrounds us. Be awake to the continually changing tones of that flow: breath as nourishment, as purification, as a tender embrace, as healing, as music, as the wind that feeds a fire, as love.

5. Be awake to the blessing of the air flowing in. Accept each inbreath as the beginning of a new lifetime.

6. Be awake to the blessing of the breath flowing out. Accept each outbreath as letting go of the old you—all those old thoughts and old feelings.

7. There are pauses in the flow of breath. Attend to them. Follow the breath as it flows into the body. Find the place inside you that is luminous if you pause for a moment at the end of the inhalation. Learn to rest in that inner center.

8. Follow the breath as it flows out of the body, and rest for a

moment in yourself, aware of emptiness, before the breath turns to flow in.

9. Just as you can be aware of the brief pause as breath turns, learn to pay attention to the space between thoughts.

10. Consider all the places in your body that tingle and glow and feel electrified when you are in the sexual embrace. Consider those moments as a glimpse of a higher reality. Then consider that every cell of your body is always permeated with that loving electricity, which is the life force.

    Revel in the delicate lovemaking on microscopic levels that is continually re-creating your body. Then dwell in the vastness of eternity as the arena for this loving.

11. Listen to the hum of your heart. It is as if a chord of music is vibrating, on and on.

12. Listen to the individual notes of a chord of music, then go back and forth between hearing the sound in its entirety and hearing the individual notes. Thus know the nature of life.

13. Listen to any sound—a waterfall, a vibrating bowl, crickets, the repetition of vowel sounds—in such a way that you merge with the sound.

    Or consider each of the vowels in turn. Chant the vowel out loud, then say it quietly, then listen to it inwardly, then listen to and feel the delicate resonance of it, then let go and listen to the silence. Notice the different quality each vowel has, the different feeling as it fades away into the resonance of space.

14. Listen to the last notes of a musical performance as they fade into silence. Be aware of that silence as the charged essence of all music. When you get that, learn to listen to each beat in the rhythm as a moment of silence.

15. Musical instruments tend to be hollow—think of a drum, a flute, or a stringed instrument such as a guitar. It is the empty space inside the instrument that is the resonant chamber. Consider your body to be a musical instrument: a delicate layer of

skin with sacred emptiness inside. Be at home in the resonance of that emptiness.

Picture every particle of creation as a tiny vibrating musical instrument, with a shape on the outside and empty space on the inside. Listen to the songs that all these instruments are playing.

16. Contemplate emptiness stretching away in every direction: emptiness above, below, to all sides. Meditate on emptiness resting in emptiness, and be free.

17. Savor how each of your senses informs you, in a different delightful way, of the play of shape and emptiness:

- *Smell.* Be outside in a vast space and stand downwind from some odor: a tree or an animal or a field of flowers. All that invisible air, all that space, and yet a few molecules of scent evoke an entire world of experience.

- *Sight.* Pay attention to light as shining through space: the space between your eye and your hand, the space between your eye and a distant mountain, the space between you and the sun. Space and light play with each other and cooperate to give the appearance of creation. Be at home in the playing of space and light. Or look at a pot and be aware of how the emptiness makes the pot.

- *Touch.* Touch yourself with a feather-light touch, then even lighter, and ever more lightly, until you cannot tell if you are touching yourself or not.

- *Balance.* Attend to your sense of balance by making tiny movements of the head. Allow the movement to become more and more invisible until you cannot tell whether you are moving. Thus be aware of the movement of stillness and the stillness in movement.

18. Pay attention to all the tiny little balancing movements the body is making as you sit there or stand there. Enter that world of movements with wonder and appreciation. Then consider that everywhere in creation, all matter on every level

is continually in a dance of making tiny or large balancing movements.

19. Think of all the heat your body generates. Be amazed: day and night you burn at about a hundred degrees, no matter what the outside temperature is. Every cell of your body is a little flame, generating heat and invisible light. All this energy comes from the sun. So in a way your body is composed of billions of tiny suns, existing within the radiant embrace of the vast Sun in the sky. Thus be aware of your essence as flame and rest in that flame.

20. Look at the night sky on a moonless night and see all the stars as discrete points of flame against a background of vast blackness and empty space. Get the feeling of how the universe is almost entirely emptiness; it is 99.99999 percent emptiness. Then love the tiny points of matter for how infinitely precious they are to shine forth in such vastness.

21. Imagine the cells of your body as being like the stars, tiny points of light in a vast emptiness. Identify with the space itself as well as the points of light.

22. Dwell for a few days in the awareness of life as flame. Track the continually changing energy tones of the flame: purifying, nourishing, energizing, refreshing, renewing, enlivening, luminous. Be free within this continuous flow of flame. Develop a tolerance for the intensity of life's flame.

23. When in the midst of passionate lovemaking, pause and savor the magical flame in your heart and in your genitals, in your skin and throughout all your senses. Together, fall into a delicious nonmoving internal movement of this light, heat, and tingling electricity. Then go deeper into the hum of the electricity. Let yourself dissolve into that resonating electricity just as you do at the moment of orgasm. Emerge from that dissolved space and continue lovemaking, but without hurry.

24. Ask your lover to tease you until you crave to be touched more and more at some spot on the body. Pause there in the unbearable and savor the craving itself; throw your awareness with

total abandon into what it is to crave. Know this delicious torment as the essence of creation. Be the vastness and emptiness craving the play and interplay of matter.

25. Reflect upon all the human passions: anger, desire, lust, greed, arrogance, envy, and any other passion that you can think of. Meditate on the different way that each is a form of flame. Let that flame take you into subtle inner flame and then into light and space, each in a different way—anger as fire and the desire to destroy something; desire as a fiery wanting to move toward something; lust as the fire of wanting to merge with something; arrogance as a way of holding the fire as if you are more luminous than some other part of creation. Be at home with the fire itself as it manifests differently in each passion. Thus learn to be illuminated, inspired, and enlightened by each type of flame.

26. Standing, surrender to gravity and let it pull you to the ground. Give in slowly. Lying on the ground, continue to give in to gravity more and more and let it pull you into its embrace. Then let gravity attract your essence in toward the center of gravity and be aware of the center of the Earth. Rest awareness in that still center of attraction around which all else rotates: the axis of the world.

27. Lie on your back in a wide open space on a day when there are no clouds. Pay attention to the vastness of the blue sky. In time, thoughts will forget to come, your body will vanish, and for a moment you will be your essential nature. Over a lifetime, come again and again to this perception.

28. As you fall asleep each night, develop little meditations you do. Lying there in bed, be aware of the flow of breath attracting you in toward your heart, and fall into the center of your heart as you fall asleep. Or lying there in the darkness, be aware of darkness extending toward infinity in all directions. Fall into that infinity as you fall asleep, and be free to play in infinite space.

29. Waking up, there is a moment of bliss when you are not awake or asleep, not in that other world or this one. Enter the quiet

ecstasy of this transitional state. Cherish it for what it reveals of your true nature.

30. Enjoy the flow of thoughts and desires through you as you would enjoy the flow of water in a river. Take delight in the flow itself. Then begin to notice the source of the river, the source of the thoughts and desires. Follow the current of desire back toward the one who is desiring.

31. Sometime when you are totally upset, stop and explore inside to see who you are. Your usual mind has been dissolved, and glimpses of your essential nature will shine through. Leave the upset behind and follow the clues wherever they lead you.

32. Become aware of what it is that you love unconditionally. It could be anyone or anything on Earth or in Heaven. Give over to that love with total abandon. Surrender to that love and breathe with the delight of it. Pay attention to every move-ment in your heart and your entire being as you love. Then be aware that for love to flow, three elements are needed: your attention, the other being, and the space between you. Love charges the space and makes it electric, full of delight. Pay attention to the way in which at one moment it is a delight to be touching the beloved and the next it is joyous to move away. Thus develop your appreciation for space itself as an ele-ment of relationship.

33. In a devoted relationship there is one current of desire that would like the love to stay the same: let this moment last for-ever, this delightful stage of relationship. There is another current of desire that says let things change, let us evolve together, let us grow closer. Let's move on. This current is a willingness to be changed by love itself. Cultivate this dual awareness of nonchange and change, eternity and transience. Return again and again to appreciating the electric tension between these opposites of adoration and detachment. The electricity itself will teach you.

34. Sometime when you are walking among other people, consider that the life in all bodies is the same Life appearing in different

forms. Silently and invisibly greet that life as you walk by each person.

35. Let go of the thought *I am this body*. Let go of the thought *I live in this particular time and place*. Let go even of the thought *I am I*.

Dive deeply into the awareness of being everywhere in all of time.

36. Feel every sensation, every touch of light, every smell, every taste, every sound as a gift to you from the divine beloved that is Life. Cultivate this awareness day by day and you will grow more intimate with life in tiny little ways. Invisible doorways in your being will open up. Attentiveness to what you are receiving is gratitude and is a gift back to life. Thus the relationship of your small being and the vastness changes, because there is a two-way flow.

37. Abandon the attitude of wanting to prolong pleasure and avoid suffering. Let the heart just be itself and feel whatever is there as it comes and goes. Return again and again to attending to the heart and its pulsations, and over time you will realize the oneness of your heart and all hearts.

38. The next time you catch yourself in a thought such as *I want this* or *I feel that*, grab hold of this "I" and perceive it by itself. Feel it through all its ranges and stages, feel into its source. You will thus experience attention beyond thoughts.

39. Wonder *Who am I?* for a minute or two and then let go of the question and dwell in the silence. Eventually a current will arise in your heart or your being, and that current will carry you into realization of your true nature.

40. For your essential Self, there is no knowledge to be gained, no enlightenment to be achieved. The Self already is knowledge and enlightenment. For the "I" that is wondering *Who am I?* there is only the ongoing adventure of discovery. There is no possibility of turning back, and there is no hurrying either. You are sailing your little boat on the vast seas of infinity and will go only as fast as the wind and currents take you. Realizing this, cherish every perception, no matter how tiny.

A daily meditation practice can be made of several of the above techniques. You might practice one of them consistently for ten minutes or half an hour for several months or years, and then move on to another technique. In addition, at odd times throughout the day you might practice a different selection for a few seconds or minutes.

As the Bhairava Tantra puts it: "Developing attention in any one or more of the ways described above, you can know, from the inside, the life that permeates us all. Knowing that life, you become friends with all. Being friends with all, your isolated 'I'-self will gradually realize its identity with the Self of the universe."

Jargon Zone (Optional, Extra-Credit Reading)

It is traditional in meditation books to have some incomprehensible jargon. If you want to learn a bit of technical talk to impress your friends, go ahead. Just don't believe that it will help you in any other way. It won't.

Here, for your edification, are a few buzzwords to impress your friends.

Chakra (pronounced chak´rah). Chakra means "wheel." Think of the spokes of a wheel coming in to meet at the center. In the human body there are places where nerves and blood vessels and glands come together. These are talked about in anatomy as plexi, as in the solar plexus.

You can tell where some of them are because they are the places in your body that buzz and vibrate if you are happy, excited, in love. What are the first couple of places you think of? Right you are. The crotch is one; the heart is another; there are several in the head. There is one solar plexus, just where you would expect an "energy center" in the body to be.

These are called energy centers because they are the places in the body that get energetic when you are excited about something. If you are thinking, it sometimes feels like the energy is in your head. If you are madly in love, it feels like the energy is in your chest, in your heart center. Or maybe lower.

The heart center is called anahata *(pronounced anna-ha´ta.) That's the place that aches when you miss someone and that gushes when you are in love.*

The sex center is a little hard to pronounce. I think that's because they wanted to make sure the kids wouldn't know what they were saying. It's four syllables, svadhishthana (sva-dish-ta´na). This is where the word dish *came from, I'm sure.*

Now, see if you can use those words in a sentence.

As in, "That babe sets me vibrating in two places, and the other one isn't my anahata."

And, "Larry, I hate to tell you this, but I want to have a purely ana-hata relationship with you."

LARRY: *"But Jane, I am feeling a certain vibration in my svadhishthana chakra."*

The last chakra we'll talk about, class, is the one you are sitting on. "That guy is a real pain in the muladhara." (It's pronounced moo-la-da´ra.)

There, you now know the four hippest buzzwords in meditation. Plus, they are fun locations in the human body.

In general, though, the more Sanskrit you know, the harder it will be for you to find your muladhara with both hands.

⊚ From Meditation into Life

At Home with Yourself

Human beings are instinctively social, and so we are oriented to the idea that wisdom comes from outside. This results in a tendency to *pave over* your innate knowing. But meditation is nothing if it is not trusting yourself, being at home in yourself. I have many friends who have practiced meditation for decades in an otherworldly spiritual tone, and they still are not at home in their personalities, their bodies, or this world. They have made a sort of lease agreement with a Hinduized or Buddhist inner world. They get to stay there as long as they observe all the proper rules and rituals. Meeting them, you would not say that they are shining examples of meditators. They seem to have given up important parts of themselves in the attempt to become spiritual.

By the way, I am one of those people who is at home in my own garden-variety Hinduism. I love the Upanishads, became a vegetarian at age nineteen, and used to burn incense all the time. I still chant Sanskrit before dawn just for fun. But maybe 1 percent of Westerners thrive on such things. When I think of the last, say, two hundred people I have worked with, I'd have to say that reincarnation, celibacy, vegetarianism, or the Hindu or Buddhist or Tibetan pantheon would be near the bottom of any list of things they needed to know.

We have good notes from Asia on meditation techniques for recluses. But we do not have such notes on what meditation is like for people who live in the modern world. The techniques are still being adapted, and Western meditation teachers are just beginning to find their voices. But that's fine, because meditation is instinctive anyway. If you do not give away all your authority, if you take a playful, exploratory attitude, you will discover what works for you.

Meditation teachers like to impose techniques on you, techniques that prevent you from discovering your own way. They know the way: just follow them. They encourage you to override your innate preferences by advertising their teachings as "scripturally authentic" and therefore of the highest authority. This lets you bypass, temporarily, the hard work of exploring your individual nature.

The problem is that meditation is ultimately about exploring your deepest cravings. The energy that propels meditation comes from your basic urges and inarticulate hankerings. When are you close to them? When some people are alone with a stereo, they put on music that reaches them deeply. Someone else might find a book, or go for a long walk and brood. How can you make yourself that comfortable right at the beginning of your exploration of meditation? The best thing you can do for your learning is to make yourself at home in meditation. To do so, take some time to recall the activities you already know how to feel at home with.

As you get a feel for what meditation is, the next step is to wrest authority away from externals and place it back in your heart. Your relationship with life is the teacher—cultivate friendships so that you have feedback mechanisms. The more you connect meditation with your passions, your deepest cravings, your unfulfilled longings, the better. Where else will you make a home for your desires? Then meditation will be simmering in your own creative fires. You won't have the Answers, but you will have energy, enthusiasm, and your own gut instincts for guidance.

All creatures have a homing instinct. They follow impulses to return to their nest. Meditation is a human homing instinct, an impulse to return to the home within yourself, and then feel at home in the world. The key is to customize meditation, be very active in appropriating it for your own use and needs, and not imitate anyone else.

Remember What You Love

Opening Your Heart to Life

Nature has designed us to thrive. Meditation is part of Nature's maintenance program for keeping us at our best. Meditation is for repair, healing, revival, inspiration, preparation for action, and love. The ability to meditate is built in, innate. It is woven into the very fabric of our bodies. It is built into the human body as part of our survival skills and is just waiting to be used.

In the same way that we have the ability to perceive a threat and become alarmed and juiced with adrenaline, we have an equal and opposite ability to perceive our own competence, to perceive beauty and safety. This results in relaxation, which lets the body recharge its batteries. These instincts balance each other and we need both. Without some sense of urgency, we are out of touch with the dynamic ebb and flow of life, and without the skill and the will to take incredibly deep repose in ourselves, we fail to discover the finer qualities of what it is to be human.

As part of life on Earth, our bodies are permeated with the adaptive wisdom of billions of years of evolution. Millions of tiny processes are at work right now in each of us, keeping the breath and blood flowing, keeping every cell suffused with oxygen and nourishment, carrying away wastes. As you read this, a dance of nerves and muscles is keeping the body balanced as the eyes move over the page, computing what the words mean, and associating that meaning with experiences you have had. When we run out of fuel, our instincts motivate us to take a break and get a meal.

The body's wisdom takes care of turning that food into the energy of moving our muscles, thinking, feeling, and perceiving. When we get tired from a long day, Nature invites us to sleep by giving us the craving to lie down and rest. A whole myriad of processes then take over that leave us renewed and refreshed the next morning, and then we want to get up and do it again. This is the rhythm of a day. And in a way, it mirrors the rhythm of meditation.

Meditation is something the body learns to crave as a way to fulfill its needs, just as it craves everything else. Just as a person might walk in the door and say, "Whew, I need a glass of wine," after that person has experienced meditation, he or she may walk in the door and say, "Whew, I need to grab a few minutes of meditation." Many people have found that meditation satisfies the need to relax much better than a glass of wine. Then after meditation, the wine tastes better. And in the morning, if we know meditation, we have a choice: go to that cappuccino bar on the way to work or grab twenty minutes of meditation. Or both. Meditation becomes part of the life of desire.

Meditation is, in fact, the main time that the body has to sort through all its desires and fine-tune them. When else do we allow ourselves to just stop and feel? It is important for our survival to know the essence of desire: that we want water, not diet cola; that we want to be loved, we don't really want chocolate ice cream; that we want to have a long conversation with our spouse, we don't really want to start a fight; that we need a long weekend or a vacation, we don't actually want to get drunk or take that drug. Desires can and often do get confused and substituted for each other. Meditation time is not at all about denying desires; it is a time to enter them more deeply, let them educate us, allow the basic impulses to connect with what is available for us now in the outer world.

Everyone who meditates has had the experience of opening the eyes after half an hour or so and having greater insight into a current life situation. Sometimes the insight comes with the kind of clarity that generally happens only after weeks or months or years. That's pretty good for something that would take up less than half of a lunch break. This has obvious survival value for people, whether they are hunting rutabagas in the primeval rain forest or hunting for a job in New York City. Yet it is as natural and instinctive as a catnap.

Unless we cultivate the attention so that we stay a little longer with these powerful experiences, we miss out on fully participating in life. The enlightenment is there but we do not stay with it long enough for it to make us brand-new. We turn away, shy of being changed. There is a tendency for these experiences to last only a fraction of a second before we leap up and are on to the next thing. This is natural because such perceptions are so impactful that we run away from them. We retreat from the intensity, even if it is intense love. But what happens then is that we feel only half-alive, if we pause at all to notice how we feel.

Meditation is the contrary impulse, also natural, to enter such a moment, prolong it by cherishing it, and thus allow it to reconfigure our senses so that we are better able to perceive life's richness at all times. When we do this, we risk being astounded and brought to our knees in gratitude just to exist.

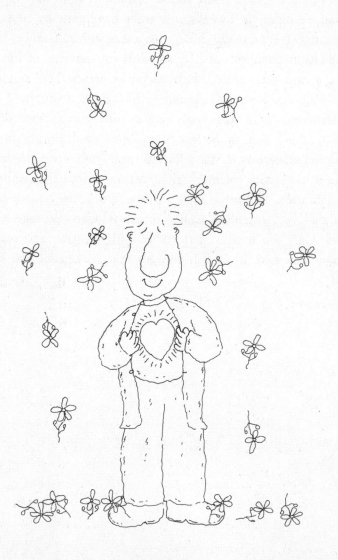

The original idea of being on one's knees in prayer or meditation is not to force humility on ourselves. Rather, it is the movement of being so in love that you are weak in the knees and almost overwhelmed by the perception of immensity. Almost everyone is afraid to enter the perception fully, because it really feels like dissolving into infinity. Each time you never know for sure that you will come back until you find yourself in your chair wondering, *What was that?* And the truth is, you are not the same person you were half an hour before. In some ways you are older, as if weeks or months have gone by, and in other ways you may feel more childlike, with a renewed innocence.

Meditation changes our contact with the essence of life. As we develop a new relationship with ourselves, we find, to our surprise, that an immense love is awakened within us. And yet there is something terrifying about such a moment of direct revelation. What if it goes away? Are we up to the task of honoring the beauty? Are we worthy? The challenge is to put your attention right into the middle of your heart to practice tolerating the intensity of love that is there. The final meditation, if there is such a thing, is to learn how to live with the richness of being alive. Can you take it? Can you take it for five minutes? Can you find a comfortable spot, breathe, and soak it in? And after you soak it in, can you get up, go outside, and spread it around?

ACKNOWLEDGMENTS

I remember being about ten years old, reading a book, and marveling at the dozens of people listed in the acknowledgments page. I thought, "How can it take so many people to write just a simple book? What's wrong with the author?" Now I know: even if the author sits alone for a couple of thousand hours to write the book, he is listening to and weaving together the voices and intelligence of everyone he has ever talked to on the subject.

Thanks to my father, for the hunts in Africa, and the many days in the ocean together. Thanks to my mother for gestating me at San Onofre while surfing.

THE SIXTIES

My gratitude to Laksman Joo for teaching me the wisdom of the Vijnana-bhairava Tantra, and Paul Reps for his exquisite translation. Thank you, Jim Fadiman for Psychosynthesis, and Ed Maupin for the Structural Integration sessions. Marshall Ho taught me Tai Chi. My gratitude to Rabindranath Tagore for translating Kabir's poetry into English. Thank you, Maharishi, for your exquisite insights into the simplicity and naturalness of meditation. Thank you, Kiefer Franz, for the Jungian dream work sessions.

Soundtrack: The Doors.

THE SEVENTIES

At the University of California, Irvine, School of Social Science: Thanks to Douglas Chalmers for the steady mentoring, to Dwayne

Metzger, for teaching me anthropological interviewing methods, Kim Romney, for his good humor and irreverent science. Thank you, Carol Knight and Acumana, for the amazing teachings. Edward T. Hall, I can hardly express how profoundly your work has influenced my entire development for the last thirty years. Thanks to Barbara DeAngelis for the many stunning conversations.

Soundtrack: J.S. Bach, The Brandenburg Concertos. The Vedas, chanted live. The Gayatri, The Shiva Sutras.

THE EIGHTIES

My thanks to Camille for her dances on all levels.

Soundtrack: Bach, *The Passion of St. Matthew.* Rachmaninov, *Symphony No. 2* in E minor. Sade.

THE NINETIES

My thanks to Camille for her immense good humor as I worked. Slayer the cat for keeping me company from 3:00 A.M. to dawn while I wrote. Thanks to my sister Dale, for encouraging me to develop my writing, and to my brother Peter, for keeping me entertained by calling at odd hours and reading to me from Churchill's memoirs and reciting entire chapters of *Bored of the Rings* from memory. Thanks to my amazing buddy Ilene Segalove, who has been immensely generous with her time and skill. Thanks to Wendy Holden for the gift of her time and attention. Thanks to Gareth Esersky, my agent, and The Twins. Thanks to Caroline Pincus, my editor, for the wonderfully humorous rock 'n 'roll email editing.

Soundtrack: David Parsons, Dorje Ling. Everything Rogers and Hammerstein ever wrote. Maria Bethania.

You are welcome to write to me with your comments and questions.
lorin@lorinroche.com

Also check out the web page for *Meditation Made Easy* at
www.lorinroche.com